RESCUED

By

LOVE

Molly Belle's Journey with Her Foal,

Promise

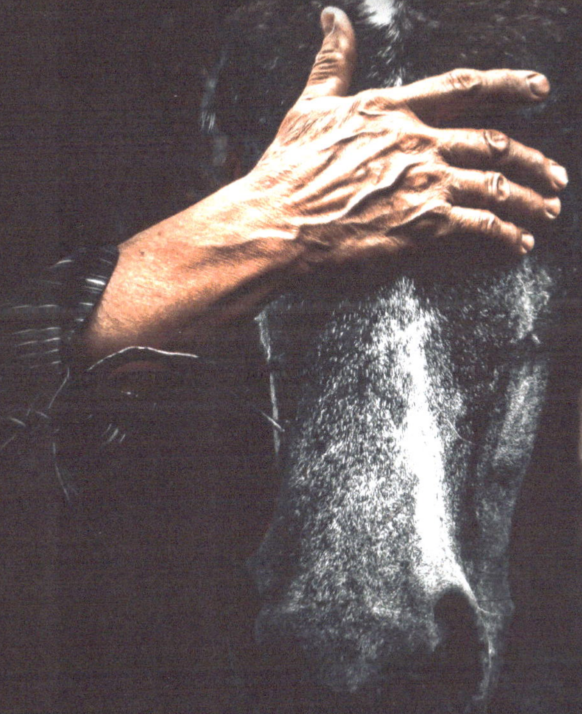

JOHN FREDERICK DERR, RPh, FASCP

Rescued by Love:
Molly Belle's Journey with Her Foal, Promise

Copyright © 2024 by John Frederick Derr, RPh, FASCP

ISBN: 979-8894799018 (sc)
ISBN: 979-8894799025 (e)

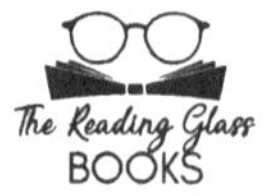

The Reading Glass Books
1-888-420-3050
www.readingglassbooks.com
fulfillment@readingglassbooks.com

PROLOGUE

Molly Belle & Promise is a story of abuse and love. It is not a typical story that you would read in a novel, in the morning newspaper or on TV. Why is this story not typical, you might ask? It is a story of a Premarin Mare and her last foal, Promise.

Premarin is a prescription required pharmaceutical with the basic ingredient being: Pre (Pregnant) mar (Mare) in (Urine). Prior to the year 2000 there were hundreds of PMU farms in the US. Today, most of the Urine is collected on a few PMU farms located outside the US. The natural pharmaceutical is slowly being replaced by a synthetic.

This is a story of grief and happiness that is being told by the Mare, Molly Belle.

This is based on a true story from the history of United in Light (UIL) Draft Horse Sanctuary.

(www.draftrescue.com)

Table of Contents

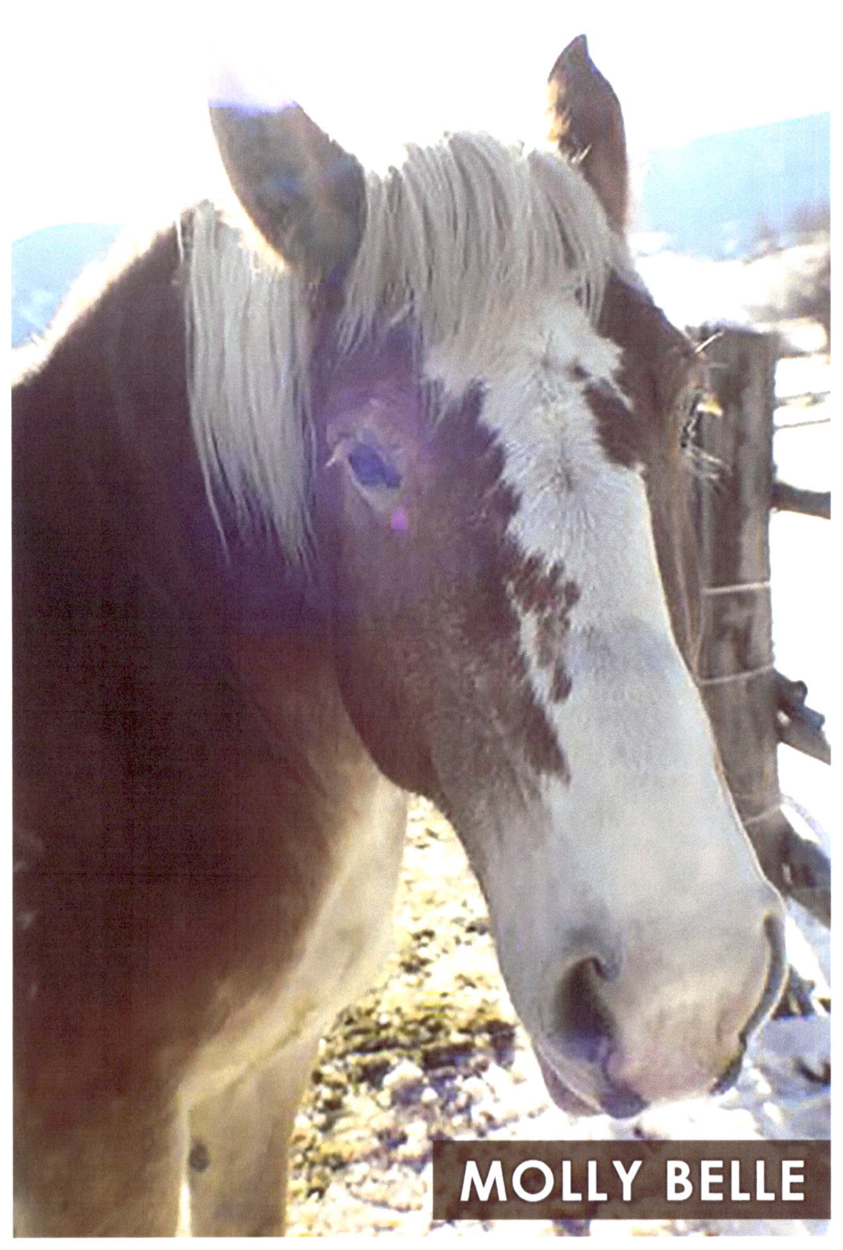MOLLY BELLE

CHAPTER ONE

MOLLY'S ABUSE

Mollie Bell is fifteen-year-old Belgian Draft horse that had spent ten years of her life on a Premarin Farm (PMU).

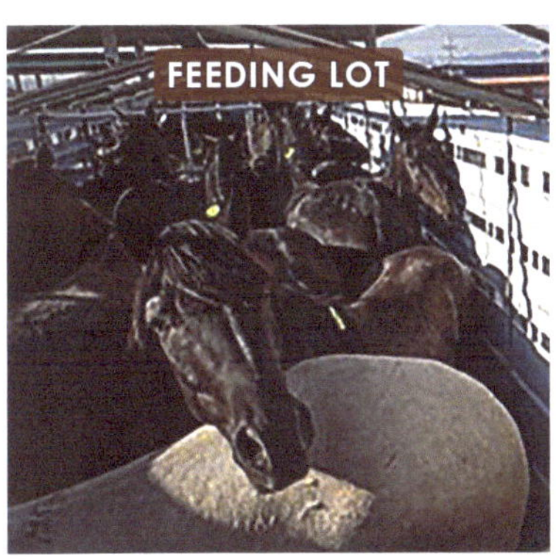

The Managers of the PMU farm determined that Molly Belle was too old to be productive and that she was no longer a valued asset to the farm!

Molly Belle's pregnant mares urine producing days were over. She was facing the standard retirement plan for PMU horses. A trip to the feeding lot to fatten her up for an additional trip to a Canadian or Mexican Slaughterhouse and ending up on the end of French fork.

On a cold and snowy day, Molly Belle was loaded and crammed into a rusty horse trailer with 20 other "non producers" to be taken to a US border feeding lot. The trip could take days without proper food and water.

This event in her life did not bother Molly Belle as much as it did the other horses. She knew that she was blessed. Molly Belle had a secret that both the owners of the PMU farm and feeding lot humans did not know. Molly Belle had a foal growing inside her womb.

After arriving at the Feeding Lot, she was herded into a crowded pen with even more horses. They were fed large quantities of stale hay to make 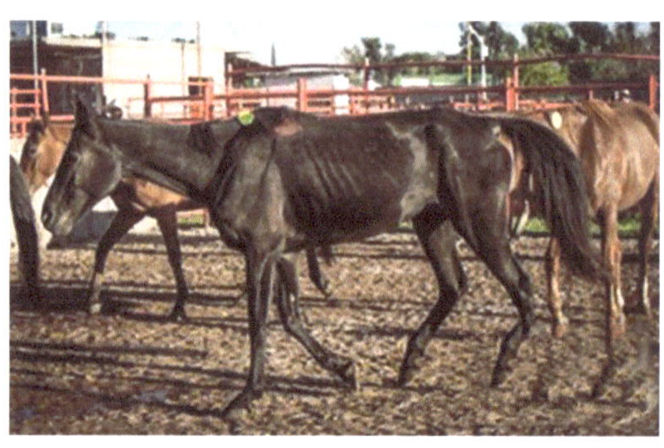 them fatter and therefore worth more money to the feed lot owners. Days went by fighting with the other horses for the rotten food.

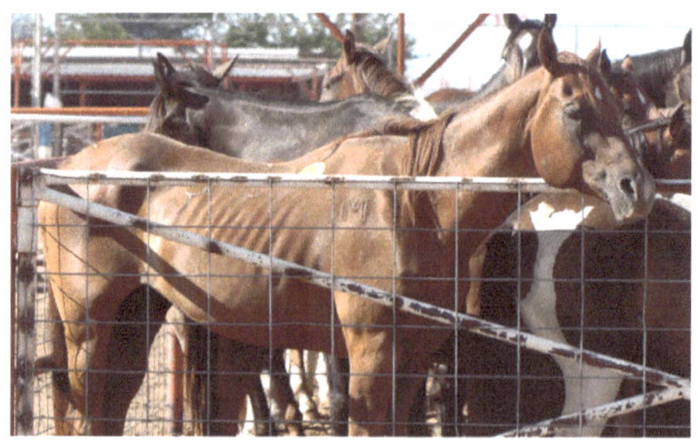 Most of the horses lost weight and their ribs began to show. She knew she was not getting the proper nutrition for her baby.

Molly Belle became more frightened than she had previously been while she was on "On Line" at the Urine producing Premarin farm.

I knew two important facts: first, I had to protect my foal and second, I had to find a way out of this pen. I was pushed hard against the metal fence by a large male draft horse. I felt the pain of the fence and I knew I was hurt and bleeding.

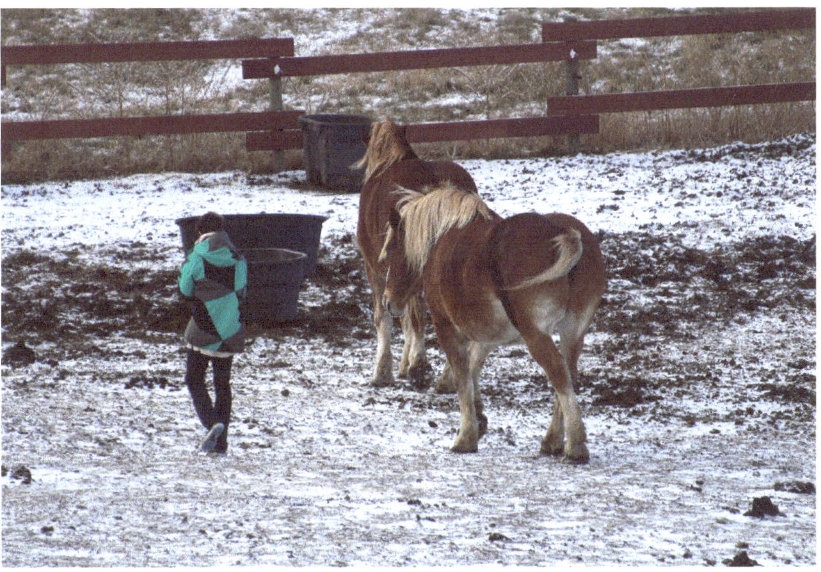

At that moment, I realized that a human was on the other side of the fence. This human was not part of the Feed Lot crew. The human had been looking over all the horses and it seemed that she was focusing on me. She was wearing a bluish green jacket. Her eyes were warm and friendly. She reached up and stroked my head. I felt an immediate connection to this human. It was a connection that I had never felt before. I knew that this human understood me and would save me and my undiscovered foal.

The human was Doctor Deb and she was looking to save one draft horse from the horror of the Slaughterhouse. Dr. Deb had space in her Montana Draft Horse Sanctuary for one additional draft horse. Suddenly, I was pushed by the other horses toward a large tent. The human followed me with a reassuring hand on the side of my head and kept whispering in my ear that: "It will be all right."

A loud human's voice announced: "The next horse up for auction is a PMU Percheron Draft Mare Number R (Roger) C (Charlie) 91." There was a loud squeal that hurt my ears.

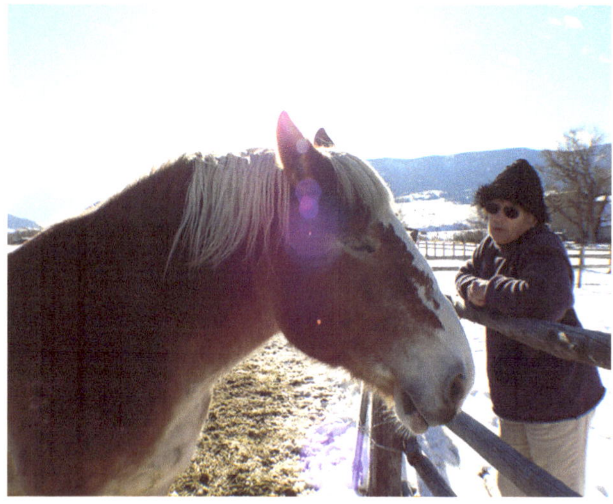

"She is a healthy mare and has been a major Premarin producer for over 10 years."

"Producer!" Molly Belle thought to herself. "That is the human metric to which I am now being measured. What about my beautiful unseen healthy foals. Am I only being measured by the urine I produced?"

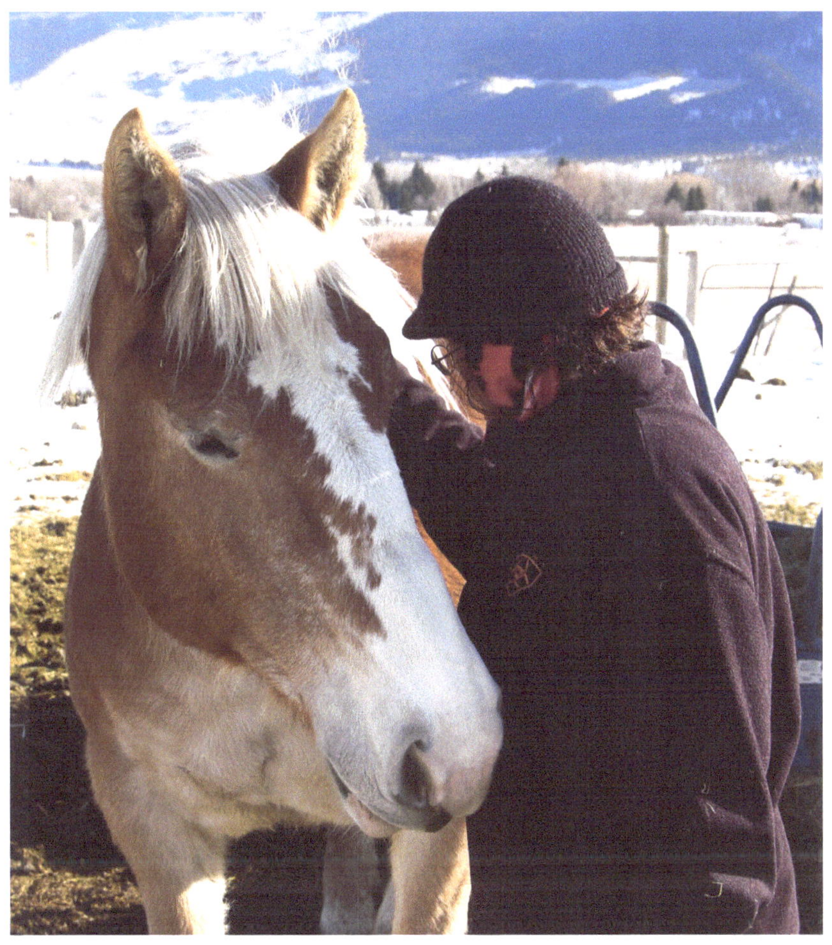

My halter was jerked, and I was led to the human with the loud voice. I began to understand that perhaps my prayers were being answered and I would be saved. Out of the corner of my eye, there was a flash of blue green jacket. It was the human by the fence. She raised her arm and was waving at me. Her wonderful voice was talking to the human with the loud voice.

The next thing I knew was that the human with blue green jacket had taken my halter and was leading me away. It seemed like a dream.

Molly Belle turned her head to look at her new friends still in the pen. "I saw that they were looking at me. Some were whinnying in happiness as they knew I was one of the lucky friends and would have a new home. The other doomed horses' eyes followed me with lowered heads as I walked to a container to take me on a ride."

Molly Belle was led to a small green container where she just fit inside. During the trip to her new home Molly Belle began to think about her past life and how she knew it was now behind her. It was a hard life on the farm but she had done what she was told by the humans and had became a good producer. The worst thing that had happened to her was the loss of all of her foals.

Molly Belle did not know how many foals she had given birth to while on the Premarin farm. After her last "On Line" cycle in the urine collection stall, she had calculated that it seemed that she was continuously pregnant. She didn't have any way to measure time. A season to her, was when she went from hot outside with many bugs and flies to a season when she grew a heavy coat of hair to keep her warm and the wet sky water turned to beautiful cold flakes like millions of white butterflies.

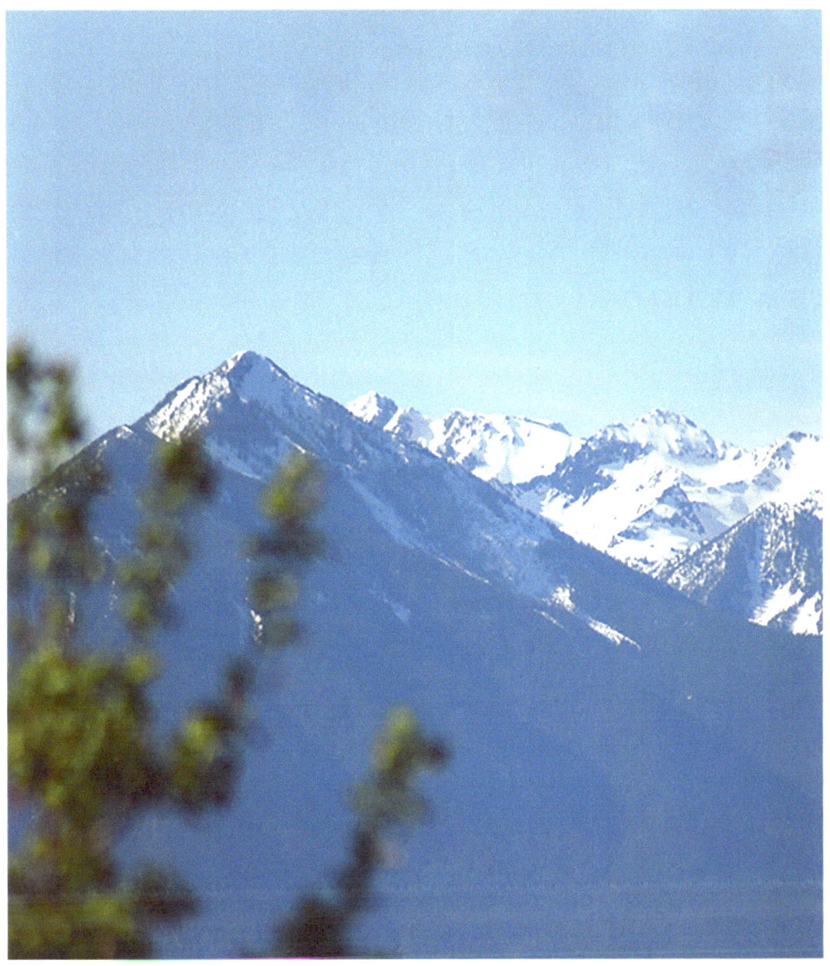

Molly Belle thought about the 10 years she had been on the farm. She remembered that there was little time between her pregnancies. She probably had given birth to at least 10 foals. When she gave birth, she never saw her foal. Her wonderful large eyes could almost see the birth but she could not quite see directly behind. The humans took the foals away and she was left to grieve their loss.

"When the humans took me back to the grass and hay, I would cry for days. Other mothers would try to tell me it was all right, but it wasn't. The other mares knew it was a sad time as they were going through the sadness themselves. Sometimes we would stand as a group and morn over our grief together."

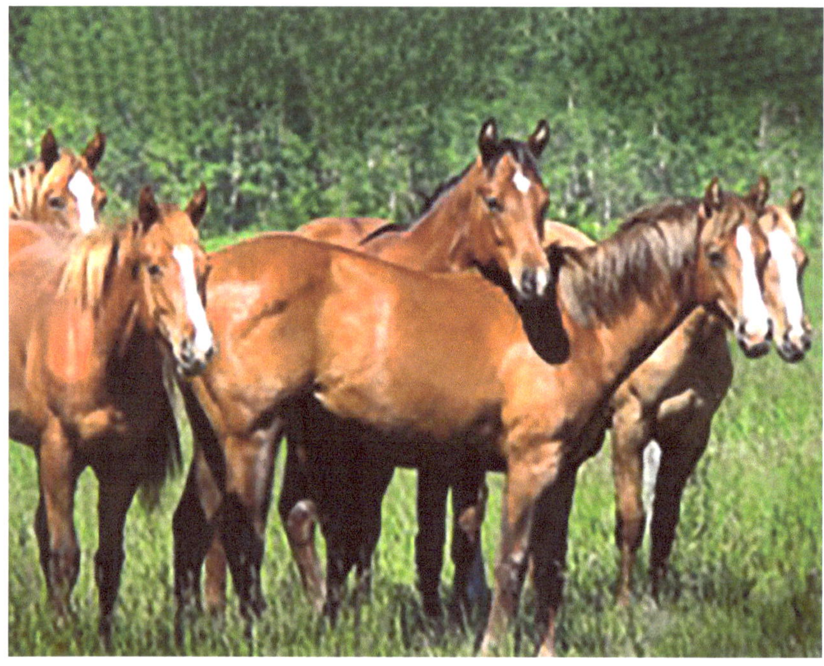

My Grieving period was short and was spent in a pasture waiting until I was visited by a stallion and I became pregnant again. Once the farm humans determined that I was pregnant, I was sent back 'On Line' in the small stall."

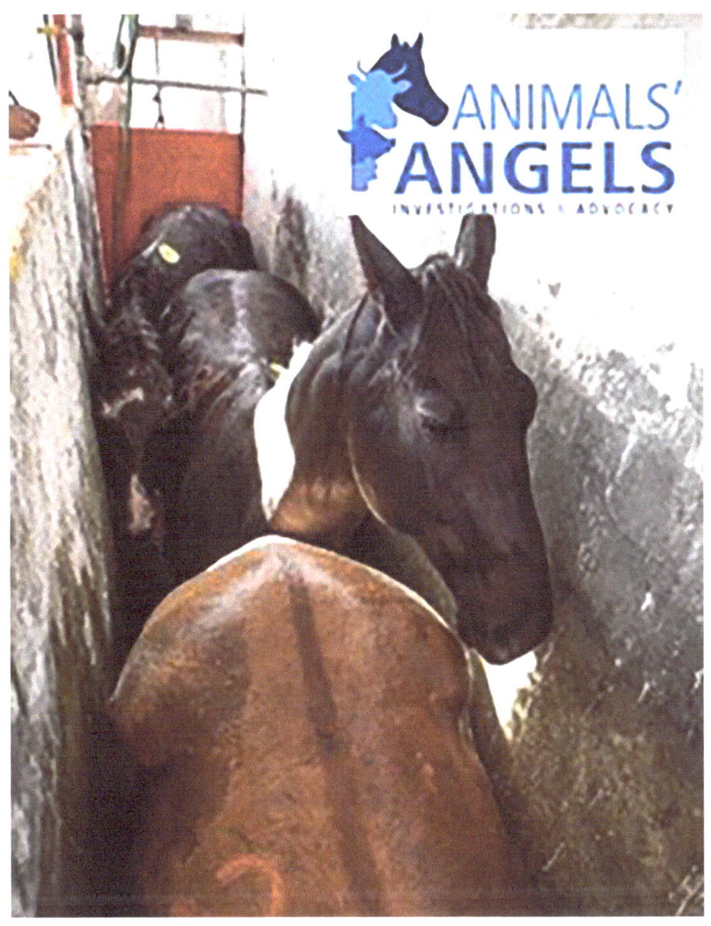

"So far in my secret pregnancy I had fooled both the farm and Feeding Lot humans. I knew the foal in my womb was not as large as in my previous farm pregnancies." Molly Belle hoped that the bad food and the traveling she had just experienced did not hurt her foal. She could feel the foal's kicking, so she knew it was still alive. She also knew that to have kept this pregnancy a secret was a blessing as many of her mare friends had tried to hide pregnancies before their trip to the Feeding Lot but none succeeded.

Molly Belle's final thoughts before the door to the green container was opened and she walked into the sunlight of the wooded and green tall Rocky Mountains was: "I have gotten away with my secret and I have a new home. I am afraid of the future as I don't know what life will be, but it has to be happier. I will be able to see my foal." She paused in her thoughts and continued in a minor panic state. "I have to take care of myself, so I don't harm my foal. And, I will have to train my foal. Something that I have never done before and don't really know how." She became restless and her panic increased.

Thus, began Molly Belle's new life on the United In Light (UIL) Draft Horse Sanctuary Ranch in Livingston, MT.

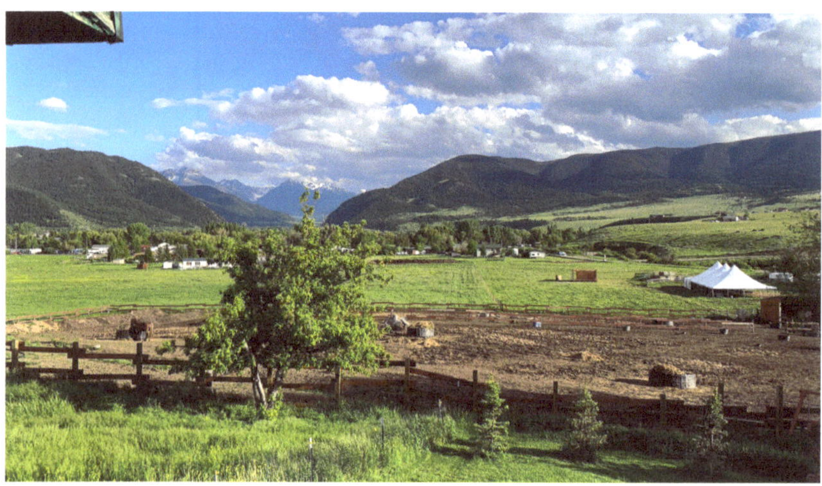

After arriving at United In Light Sanctuary, Molly Belle was led to the Ranch's Elder Pasture where she was going to be introduced to her new friends. The other horses were in the Main Pasture. They came up to the fence to meet her. Molly Belle didn't really know what to do. She was now in a strange place with strange horses. Panic took over. She ran to the end of the Elder Pasture and ran back to the gate looking to try and get back in the container.

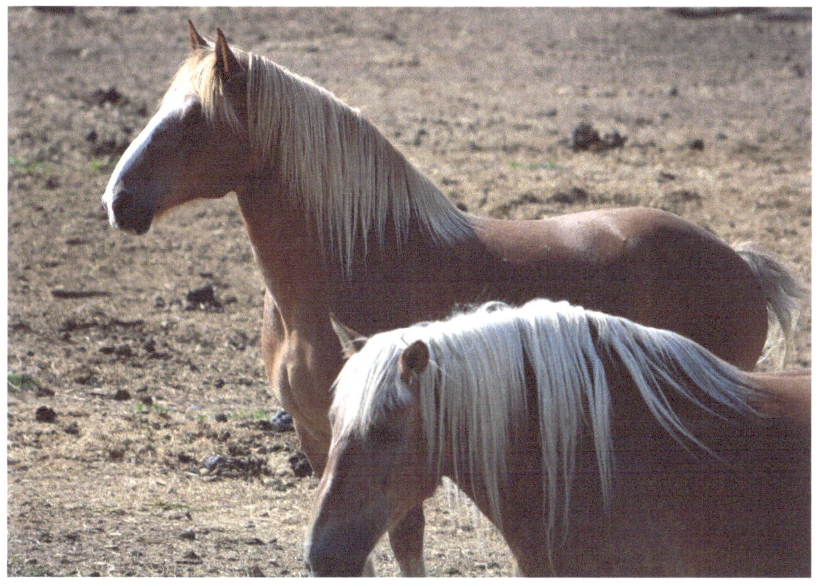

She found that now the gate was closed. She turned and ran back to the other end of the pasture. What was she to do? She stopped and looked across the fence and saw the other horses staring at her. This did not help her panic. She continued her galloping back and forth until she was too tired to move.

She couldn't eat or drink. But, what was she to do? She could not calm herself. Her state of panic went on for two days.

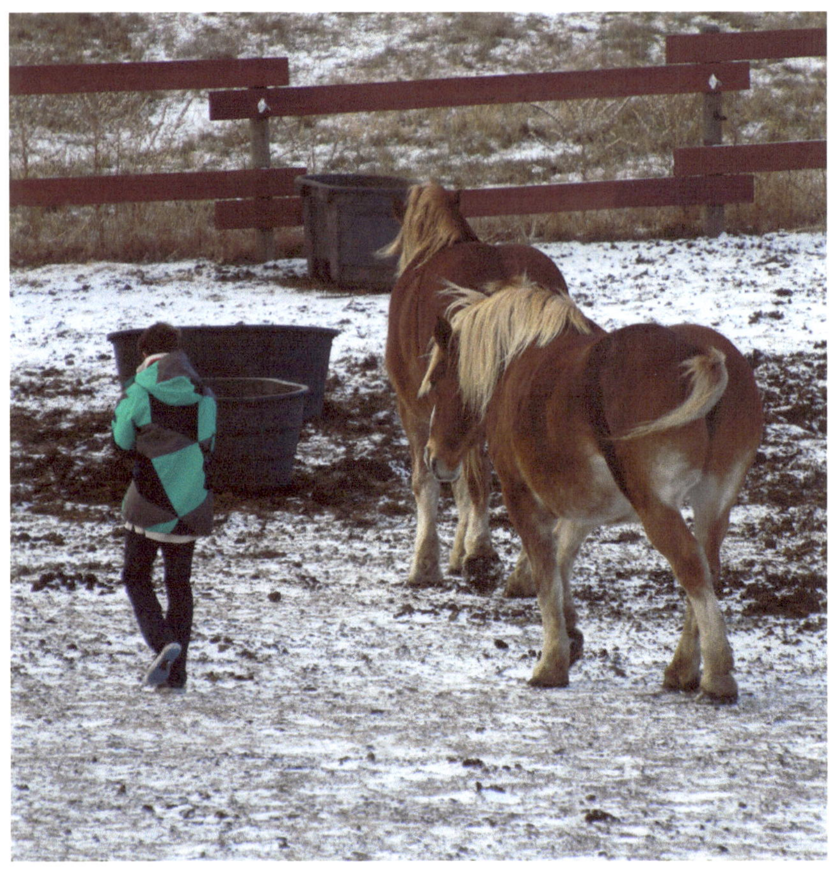

Then on the third day as she was standing in the corner of the pasture, she saw the human with the blue green jacket of the human that had helped her to escape.

"The human was walking slowly towards where I was standing. I felt the same calmness I had felt in the Feeding Lot. I heard that musical voice tell me: 'It will be all right.' "She said those wonderful words over and over again. I became calmer and bowed my head."

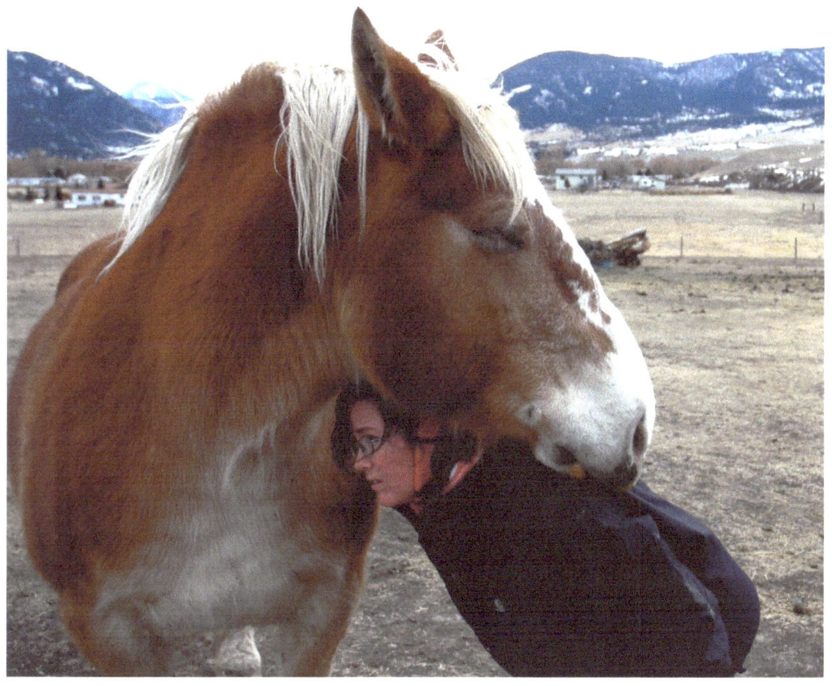

"I am Dr. Deb and you are at my ranch." She said: "You will be alright, and I am going to help you. I am going to tell you about Knight of Dreams." Dr. Deb had left the gate open. A large white Percheron draft horse had followed her into the Elder Pasture and was slowly walking to where Molly Belle and Dr. Deb were standing.

Dr. Deb rubbed Molly Belle's head and said: "I would like you to meet Knight of Dreams. Knight was my first horse and has been my friend for a very long time. Knight was abused by his owner until I brought him here."

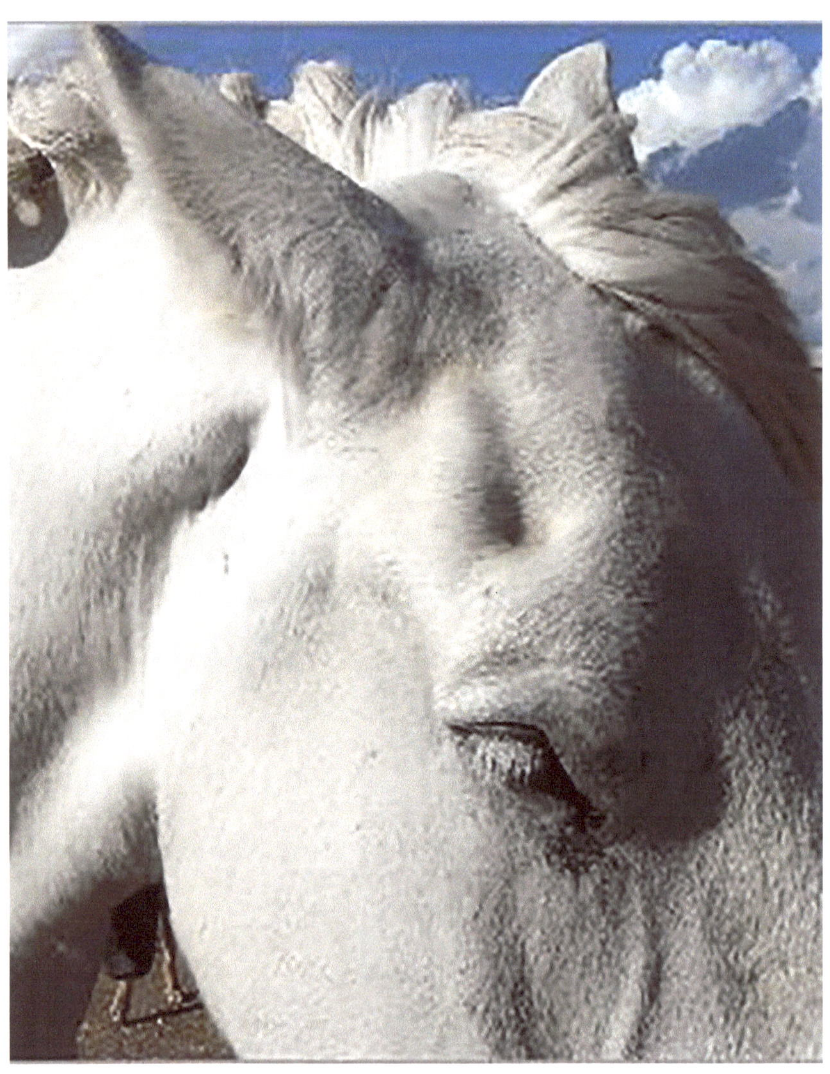

"Knight has been the leader of the UIL Herd for many years. He will help you to become a member of the family of friends and to be unafraid. I am going to leave you with Knight while I look after the other horses." Dr. Deb left the pasture where Knight and Molly Belle were standing.

Molly Belle looked over at Knight and determined that he was one really big horse. She said to herself: "I am a little afraid and I am not sure I am safe or not.

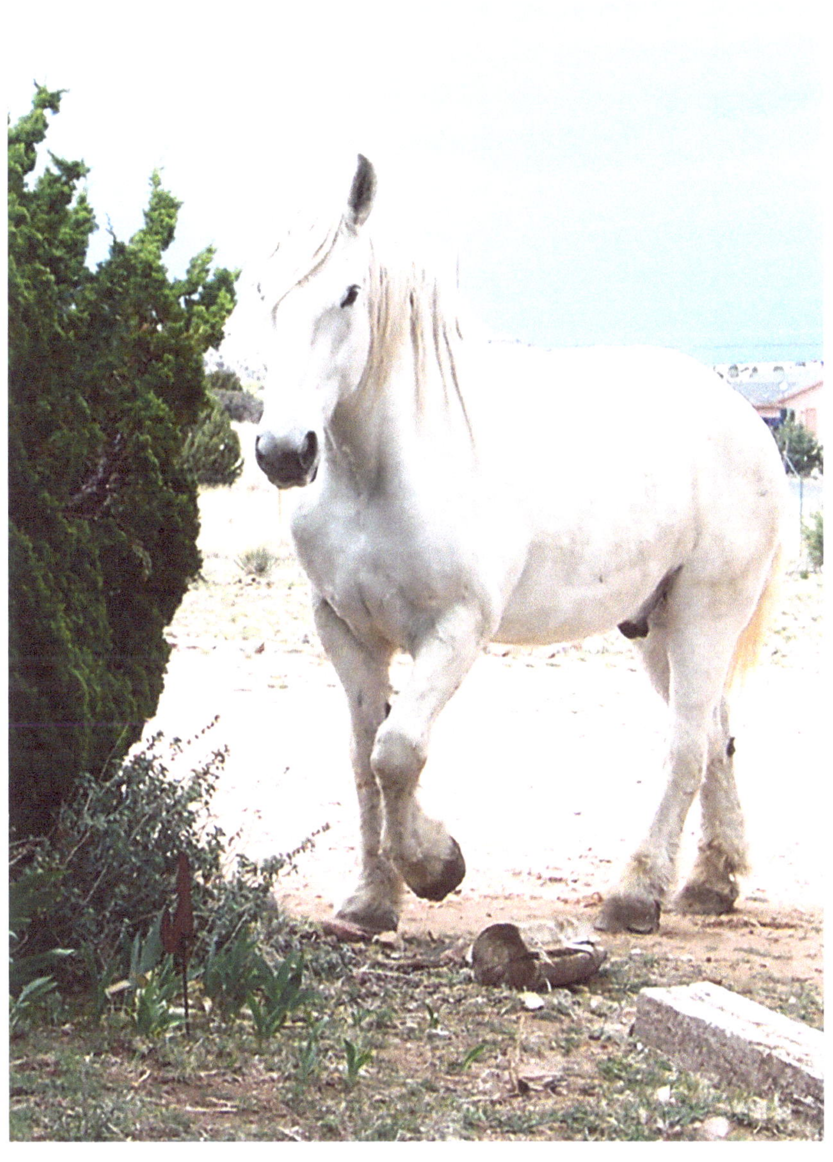

The only large male horses I have stood next to wanted to make me pregnant and back On Line as soon as possible."

"I started to regain my panic state and bowed my head and tried to get control of myself. I felt a tender nudge. It was Knight providing me with the assurance that I was safe. We stood together in the corner of the pasture for a long time. So long that the other horses who had been watching grew tired of waiting to see what would happen and they went back to eating hay.

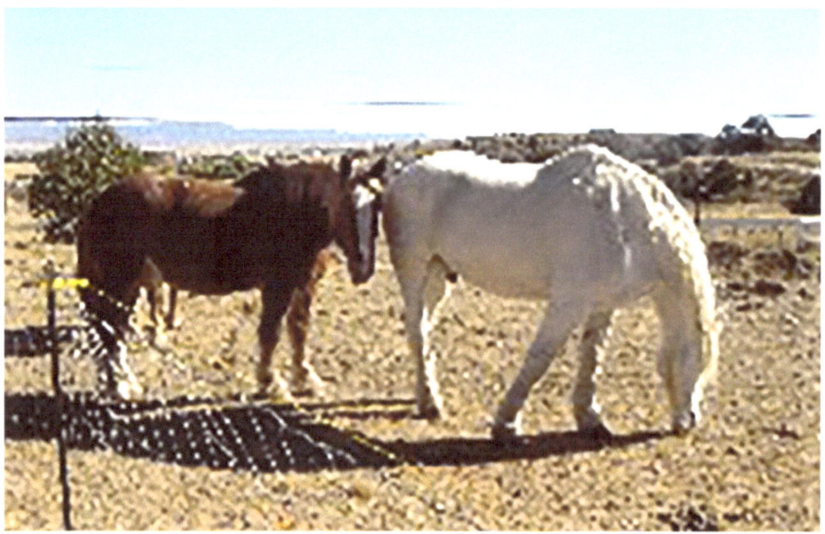

I felt another nudge on my backside pushing me forward. Knight was urging me to move outside the elder Pasture to where the other horses were standing. He continued to nudge me through the gate and up to the hay feeder.

The horses that were already eating moved aside so I could eat." For the first time at the UIL ranch, Molly Belle started to eat the enriched hay. After her first bite she stopped and moved slightly back. Knight must have thought she was going to leave and was about to nudge her back to the feeder. Molly Belle whinnied: "I was not leaving I have never tasted hay that was so sweet."

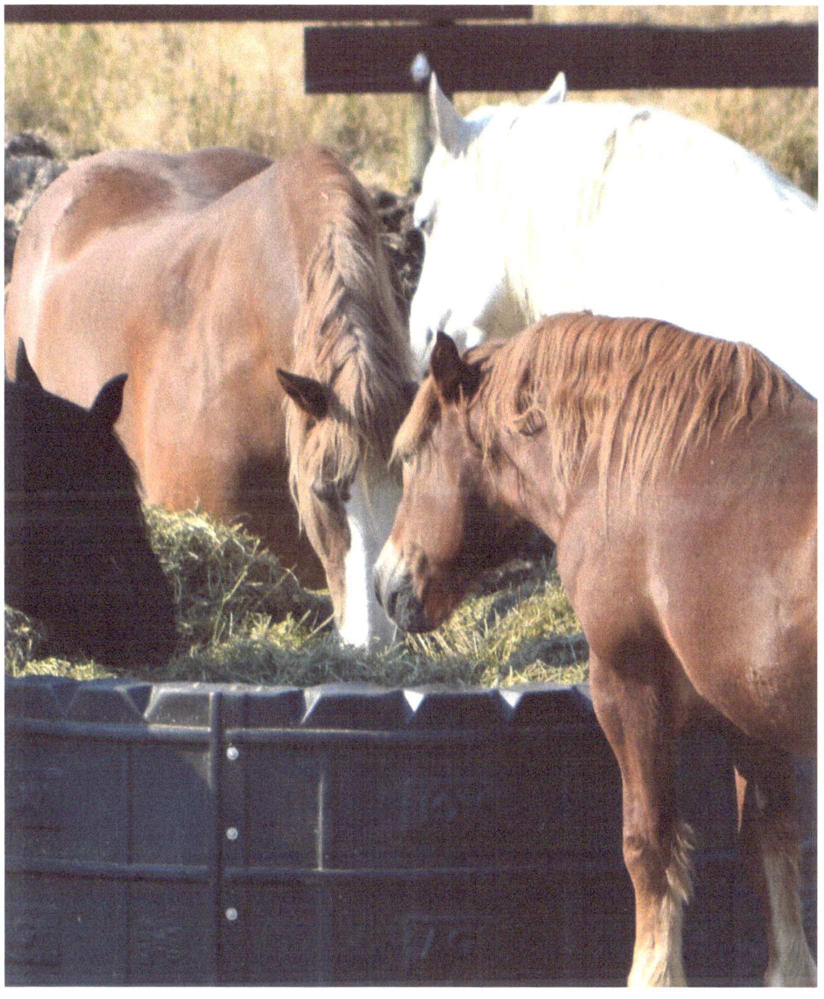

"After I had enough hay, Knight nudged me to the water trough where I drank deeply the spring water that flowed through the UIL Pasture." I thought: "This surely must be a dream. Maybe that is why my new friend is called Knight of Dreams."

Knight helped her over the next few days. Knight's thoughts overwhelmed her as he knew by her sweet musky odor that she was with foal. Knight continued to encourage her to eat and drink to help her foal.

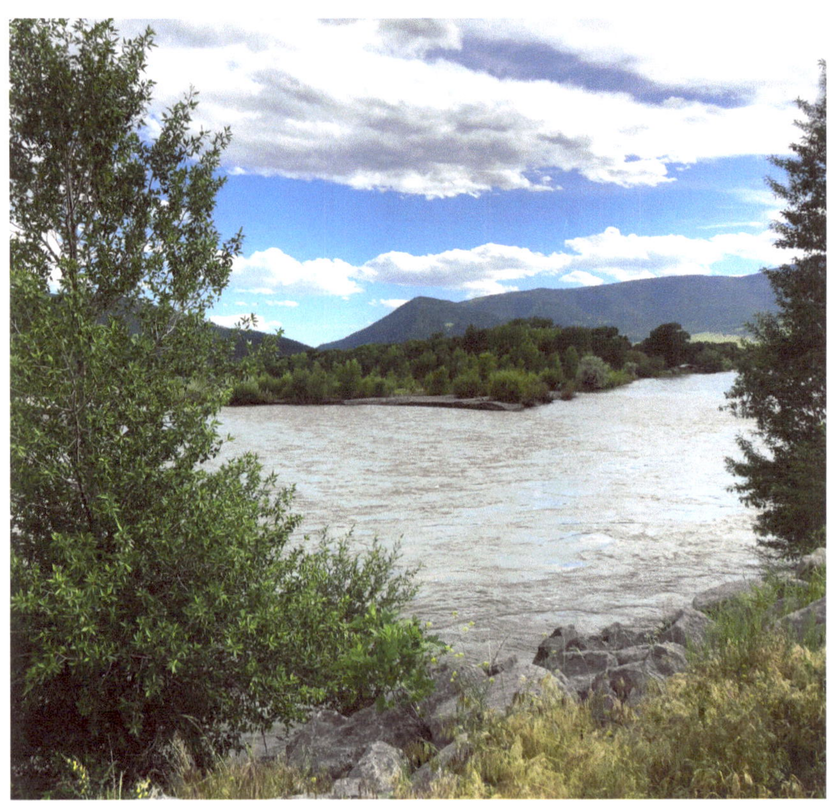

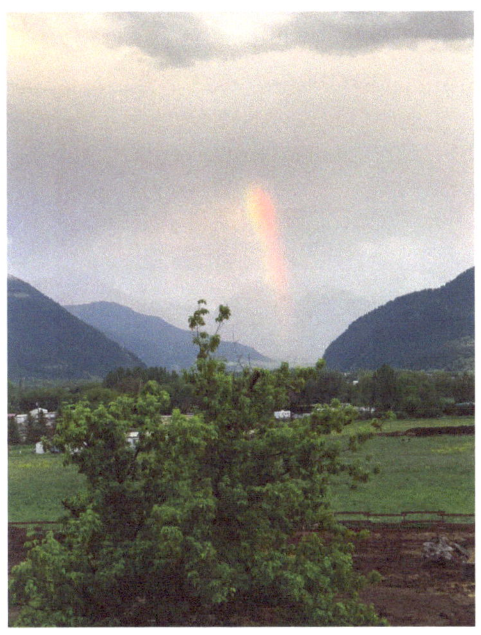

Slowly Molly Belle regained her strength, and the horses began welcoming her to the herd by touching noses in greeting. At times there was a great deal of whinnying.

"I now had my own hay, and I was able to trot around the pasture. It was warm and there were dusty patches of ground.

"I was able to lie-down and roll on my back in the dry earth while kicking my legs in the air." Molly Belle whinnied: "Freedom".

The next day after a hardy meal, Molly Belle suddenly stopped dead in her tracks: "What about my baby, I have to be careful." She stopped trotting around the pasture and rolling in the dust. She slowed down to a steady walk.

The additional weight of her foal caused her to walk funny.

She began to worry: "I must not show Dr. Deb that I am pregnant. Maybe she does not want a pregnant horse." I bowed my head in worry: "Maybe Dr. Deb will send me back!"

She panicked and kicked her hind legs in protest. She again began running back and forth along the fence line. Her suddenness scared her new friends. They ran from where they were grazing to the far end of the pasture. That is all the herd except Knight.

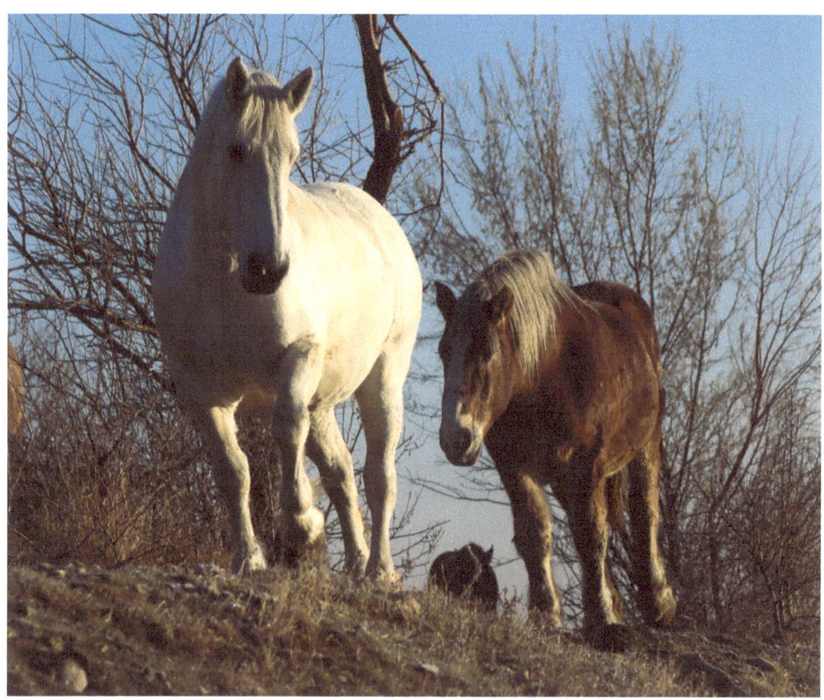

Knight ran after her and cut her off making her stop. Knight gave her a loving nudge and she felt his concern.

Knight sent thoughts to her and assured her that she was not going back to the bad place.

Molly Belle thought: "I have new friends and a place to run. I am pregnant and will witness the birth of my foal. I have the opportunity to raise my foal to be a fine horse. The humans will not take away my foal. I should be thankful, and I should not run around like a crazy horse."

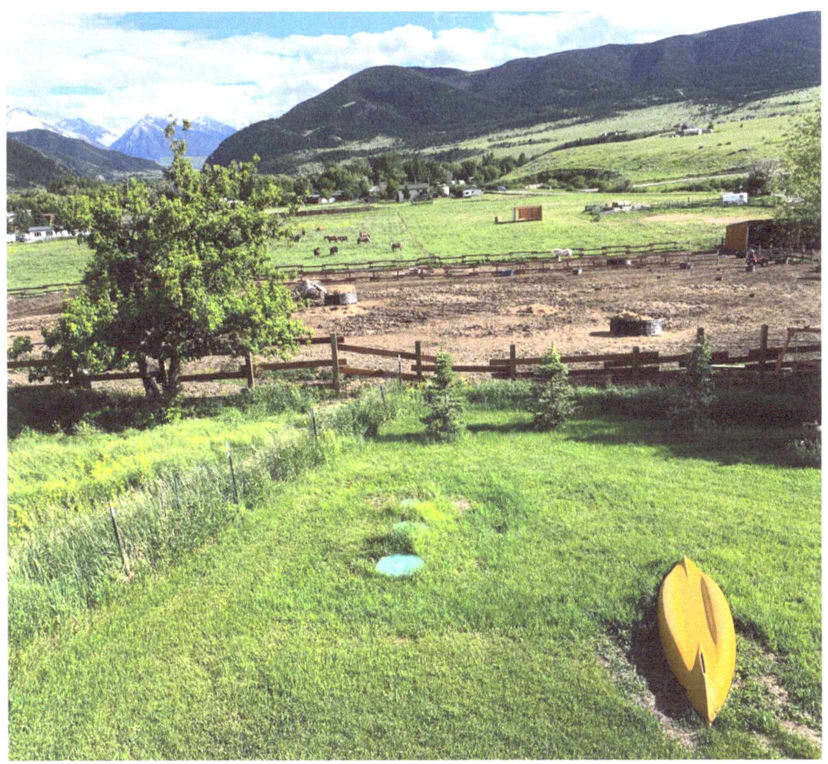

The next few days were spent calmly as Molly Belle explored the ranch.

She learned that all her new friends had also spent time in a bad place and Dr Deb had brought them to this place to enjoy life.

At the ranch there was no work for the horses. Dr. Deb felt that her horses had worked very hard all their lives. They had endured both physical and mental pain and now they were retired and could live out the rest of their lives in happiness.

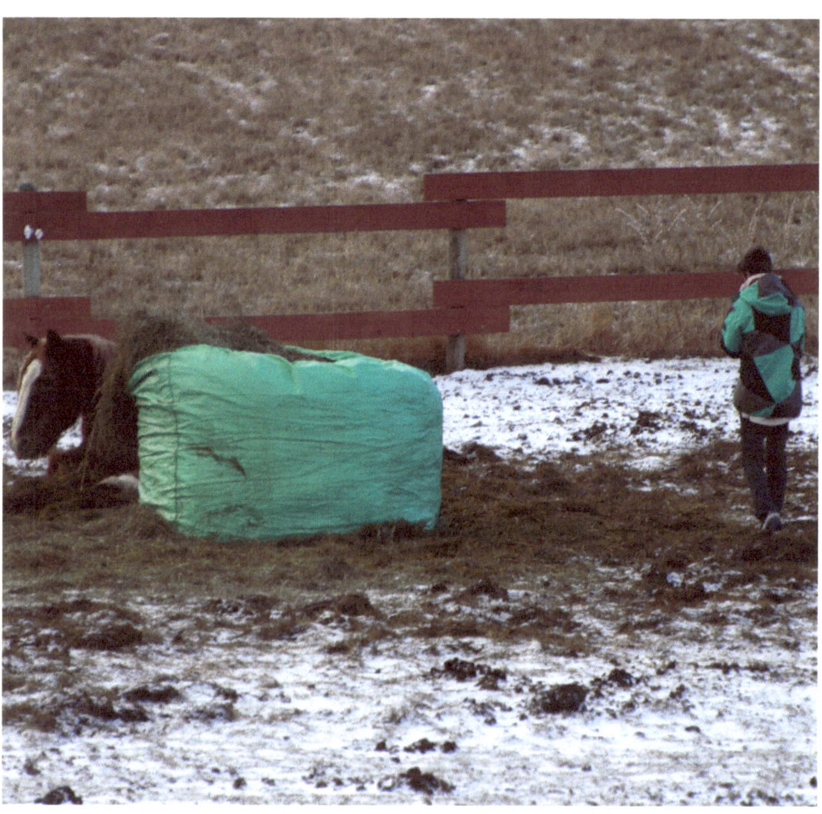

A couple of days later, after I had my fill of eating sweet hay and was laying in the sunlight , Dr. Deb came to see me.

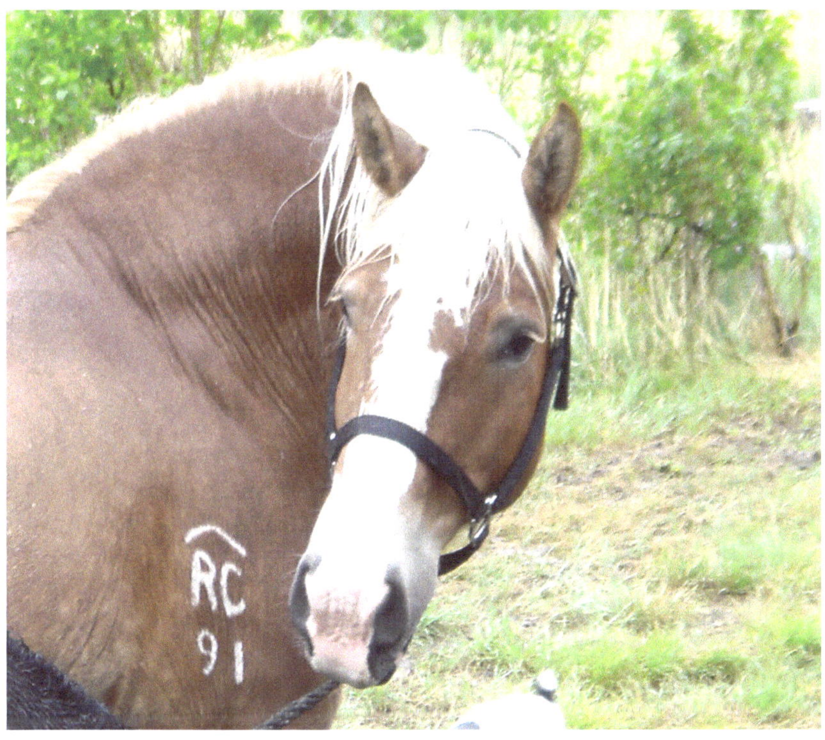

She smiled and looked directly at me. She rubbed my head and said: "I don't know your name RC 91. From what I know about the PMU farm they don't give or understand their mare's names. They probably just called you RC 91."

Dr. Deb paused and said: "Is that Right?"

Molly Belle **whinnied** as loud as she could in response.

"I sure wished I could talk to Dr. Deb. Some humans understand me more than others. I remembered at the farm that a small young human used to visit me when I was grazing in the pasture. He would spend a long time brushing me and talking to me."

"I would whinny and he seemed to understand without either of us making additional noises. I would move my head back and forth as well as up and down. I also let him know what was good or bad by raising or lowing my ears."

Dr. Deb continued: "There was nothing in your papers on your name except RC 91.

"Is that what you want me to call you?" Dr. Deb paused "I don't think you want to be reminded of your time on the farm."

Dr. Deb spoke again: "I will say some names that seem appropriate to determine whether you like any one name better than another."

I bopped my head up and down and tried to get Dr. Deb to understand me and that I wanted to tell her that I wanted to be called Molly Belle.

Dr. Deb started speaking names. I did not like any of the names and I showed my dislike by pinning back my ears.

All of a sudden, she said: "Molly Belle".

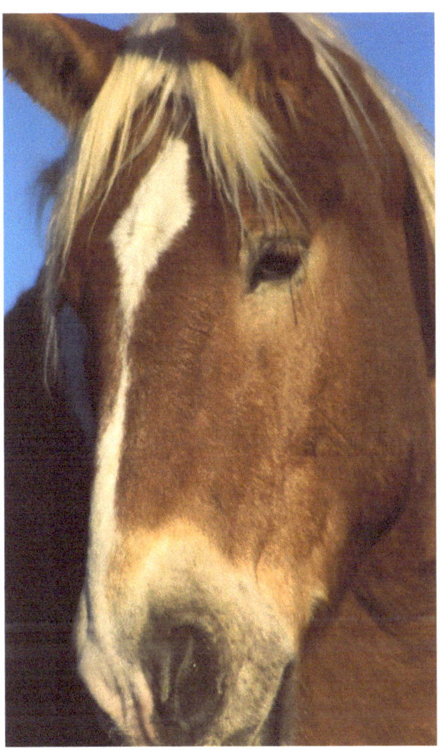

I went crazy but not too crazy as I did not want to scare her. I perked up my ears and whinnied.

Dr. Deb figured it out and said: "That is going to be your name, Molly Belle."

She continued: "Molly Belle, welcome to United in Light."

The naming session was followed by many days of Dr. Deb and other humans checking my feet, teeth and other parts of my body that I do not wish to speak. It was at this point that Dr. Deb discovered that I was pregnant. I remember it clearly and at the time I almost panicked again.

She was checking my health when suddenly she stepped back and exclaimed in a loud voice:

"Molly Belle, you are pregnant!"

She went on: "How the devil did you hide your pregnancy from the farm and feed lot humans?"

I was so afraid that Dr. Deb would not want me anymore.

I panicked. I started to run along the fence trying to get out of the pasture and run away. Back and forth I ran rubbing the fence and cutting myself. Dr. Deb ran to catch up to me, but I was too fast. Back and forth and in a circle I ran. Dr. Deb yelling at me that it was all right. My ears were so flat against my head they hurt. Finally, I realized I was not going to escape, and I suddenly stopped. I stopped so unexpectedly that Dr. Deb bumped into me.

My whole body was shaking, and I was sweating from the run. I was really scared. All the times at the farm when things looked bad, I had been scared but I just accepted the bad. But today, I had experienced both freedom and love. There was no way I was going back to the bad.

Dr. Deb was quiet and just kept rubbing my head and telling me in a calm voice: "Everything is going to be all right and it is all right for you to be pregnant. We will all love your foal."

Then Dr. Deb stepped back and looked at me right into my eyes and said: "Molly Belle, I can understand your fear of losing your foal. You have lost so many foals that it is hard for you to understand that this time you will be able to keep and take care of your foal. You will be able to nurse your foal, to teach, and watch it grow into a fine horse.

"Don't be afraid. All our humans are also your friends. Your new horse friends love you and will welcome your foal."

"Please understand and don't be afraid."

What wonderful words Dr. Deb spoke to me that day. I even felt my foal stir inside my womb. I thought, no more hiding or going into a fear panic. It is a time of happiness and love for my foal and all my new friends.

During the next few weeks everything was a blur. Dr. Deb and her friends were always with me. Other humans came and checked out my foal to make sure that both my foal and I were okay. It was a wonderful time in my life. The bad time and the other missed foal births in my life were forgotten. I felt blessed.

CHAPTER TWO

THE LOVE OF PROMISE

It was a lovely warm evening when I felt my foal start to stir and give me indications that it was time. I wanted my foal to know that it was going to leave the security of my womb and join the outside world. It was going to be with okay with me and our new friends.

Dr. Deb and the other humans were continuously watching over me and they could see that something wonderful was beginning to happen.

It was early one sunny and warm morning when I knew it was my time. I went into the pasture and found a large patch of soft green grass and I laid down. I was just going to push and let my body do what was necessary to give birth to my Foal. This time I was not going to be standing in a small stall and harnessed to the wall so I would not move. No farm humans would be pulling my foal from my womb.

I was in a euphoric dream as I gave birth to my foal. Dr. Deb assisted as my foal emerged into this beautiful world. I had given birth to a beautiful midnight black male foal with a white spot on his face.

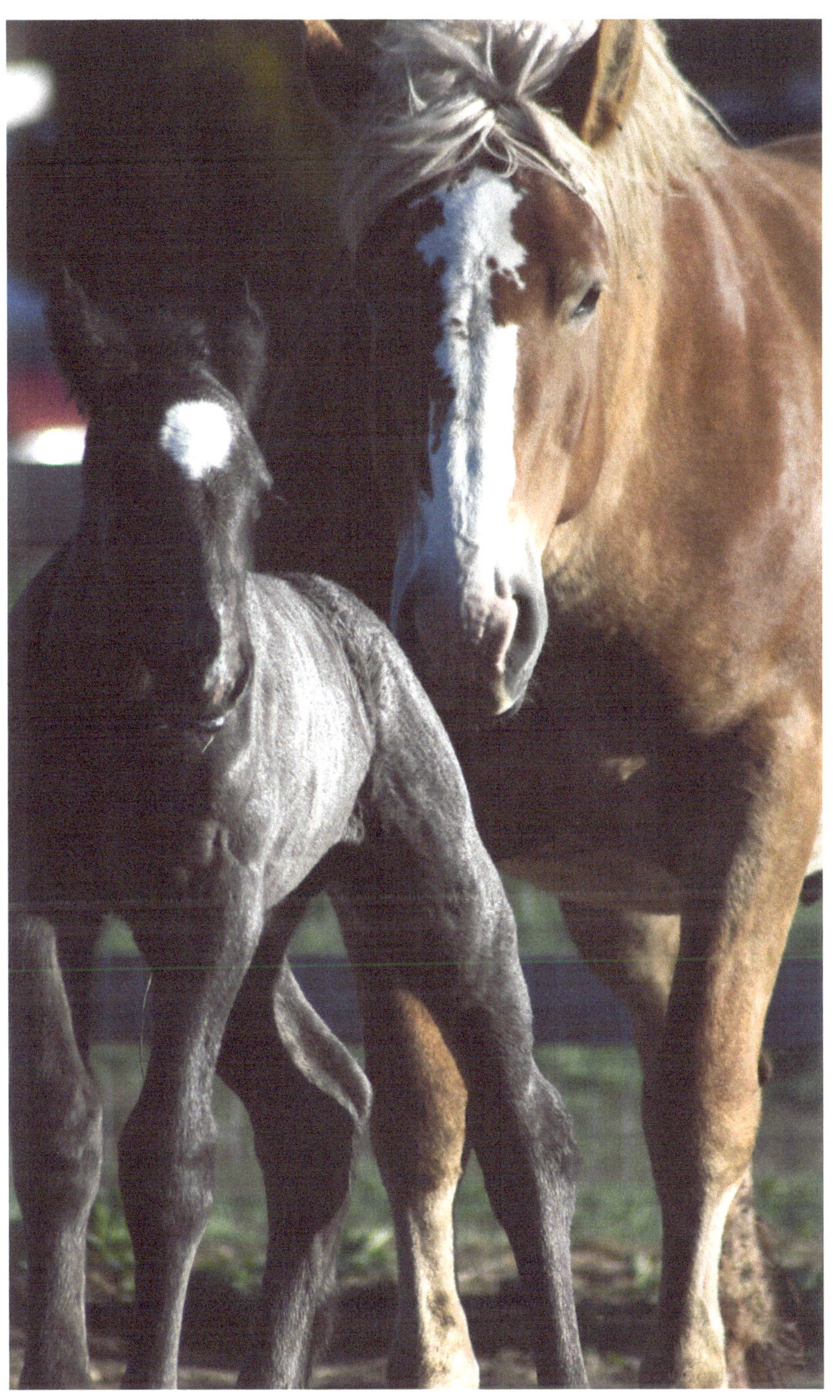

I was a little dizzy and I thought: "The bad times were over."

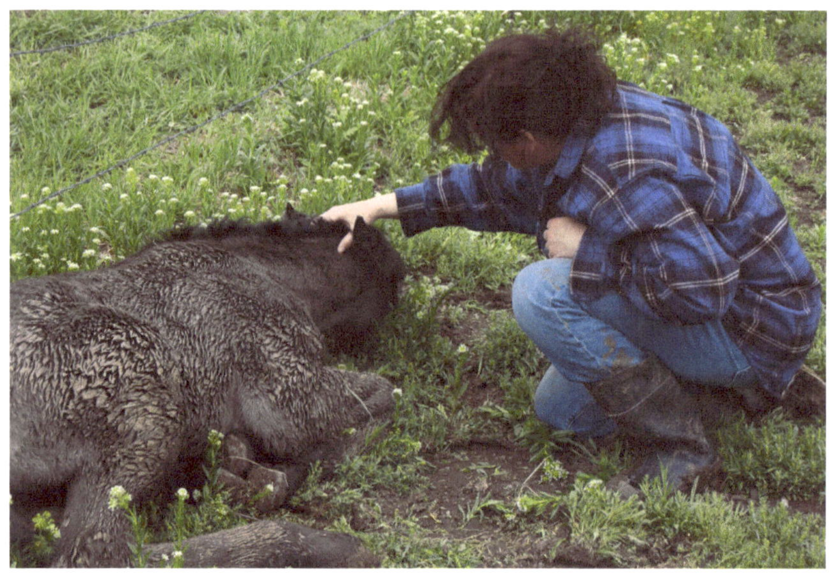

I was surround by friends and a beautiful foal. He was at my side stirring with life and looking to where he would find the nourishing milk my body is now producing.

While I was cleaning my new foal he started to move. His spindly legs were moving back and forth as he was trying to stand up. I made my foal a promise that he would live.

Dr. Deb looked at me and rubbed my head. Almost in a synchronized thought we said:

"He will be called,

PROMISE."

There began a chorus of whinnying and the humans cheered.

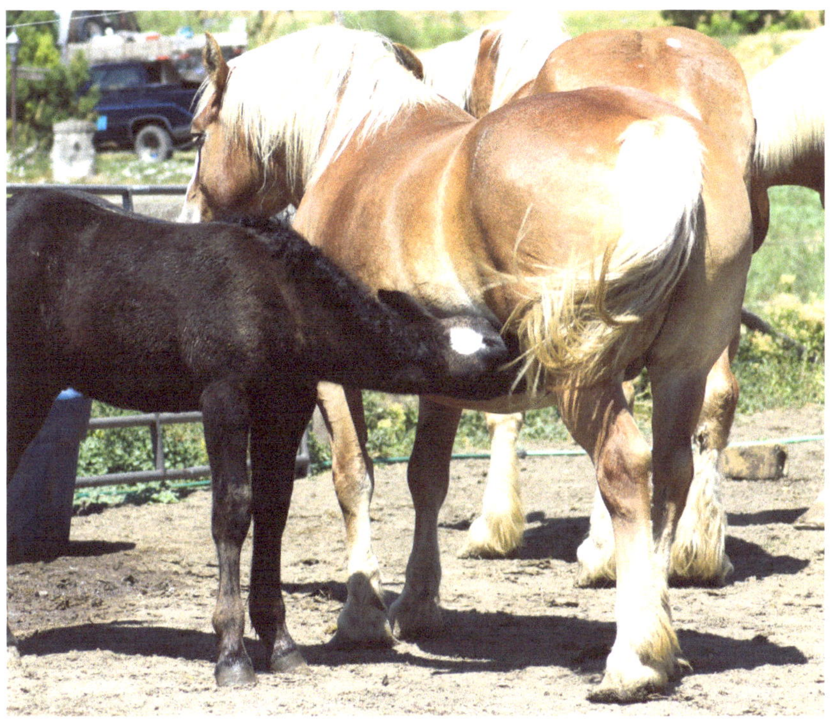

I stood up so Promise could stand and seek out his nourishment of my milk. The sun broke from behind a large Montana Blue Sky Cloud and made shadows of us.

Days went by rapidly as Promise grew and I was able to be a Mom. He would romp around but not too far from my side. We were a pair. Every one of the other horses were substitute Mom's or Dad's. The humans could not get enough of Promise and with his love, he made sure they would want more.

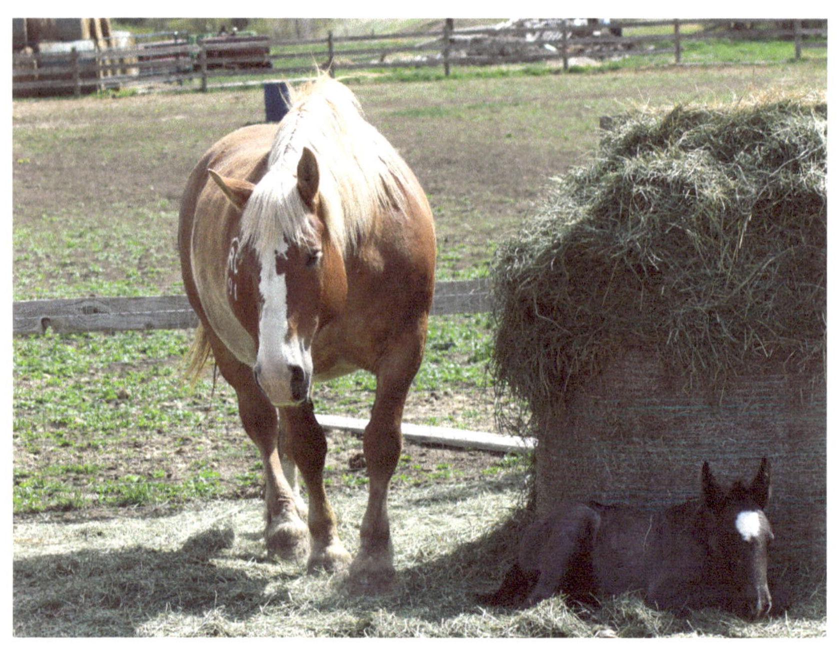

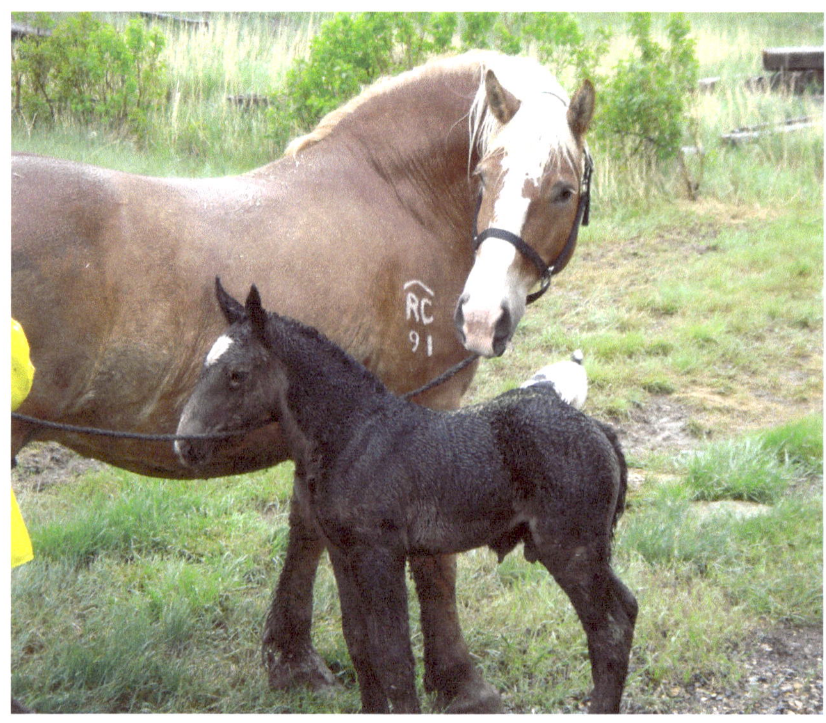

What can I say: Promise was a beautiful foal! His coat was a glowing dark satin black. The whiteness of the hair on his muzzle was in deep contrast to his black coat. You could always identify Promise when he took a run at you. His white spot on his head was like a headlight coming out of a dark tunnel.

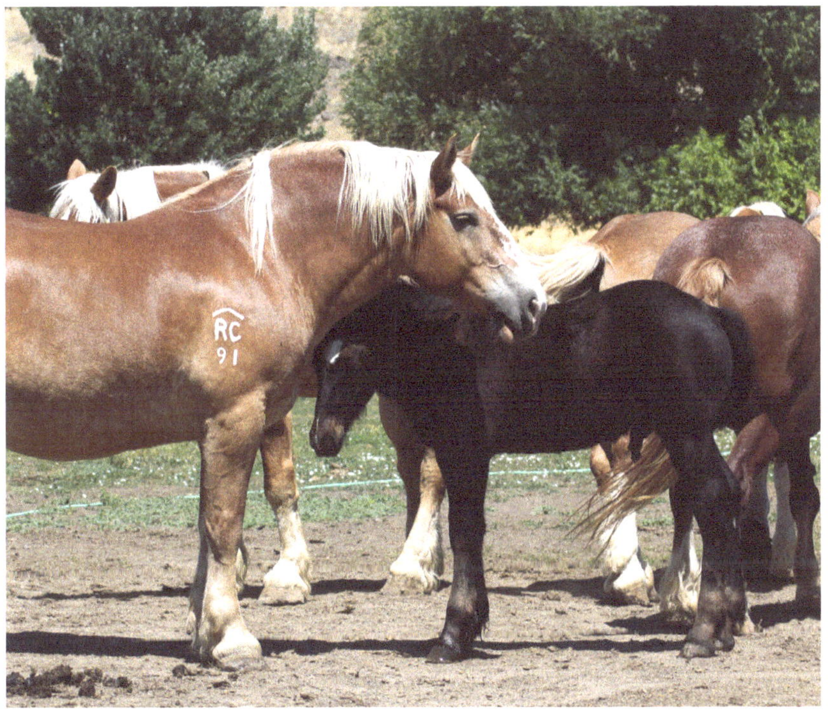

Promise was an inquisitive colt. After he had his fill of milk, he would lie down at my feet and take a nap. Sometimes I would join him, and we would lie together in the sun just resting. No worries. Just a Mom and her foal. Friends would come by and nudge us, and we would understand their love.

Promise and I would meld our thoughts together as we rested. He would ask me questions about how I grew up and who was his father. I would lead his thoughts to ask a different question. One that would not have to be answered with stories of the bad times. As he grew older it became harder and harder to avoid questions of his birth.

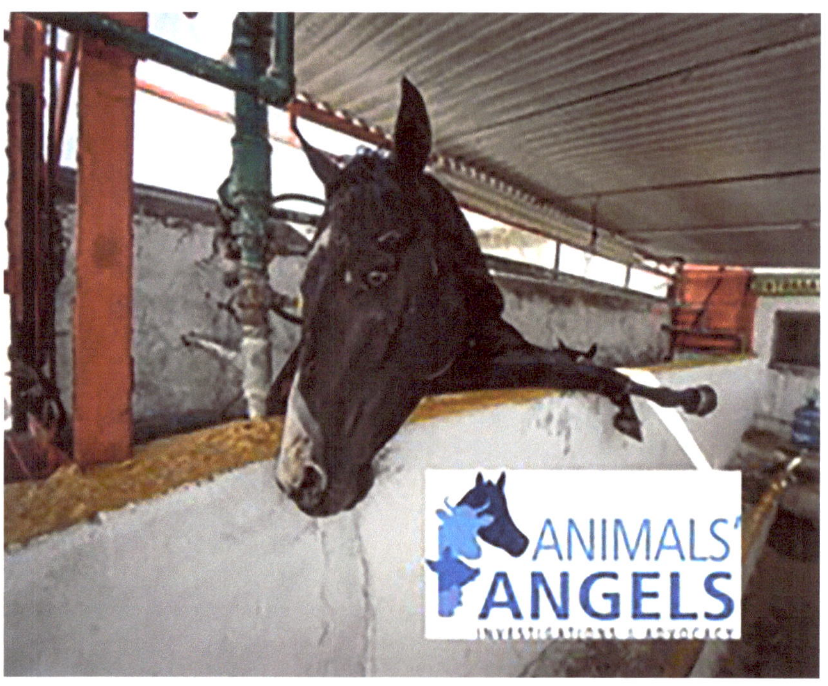

I began to tell Promise about those many years of my time on the Premarin farm and standing in a small stall all hooked up with tubes and bottles. At first Promise did not understand what I was talking about. Urinating was such a normal thing to do and to do anywhere he felt ready to go.

Gradually he began to understand that Mom was forced to stand in one place because she was tied to that small stall with rope. It finally dawned on him that when his Mom was growing up, I was not free to run, jump and play. He learned the definition of work and the difference between work and play. This was very confusing to him and he went to the other friends in the herd and asked them about work and play.

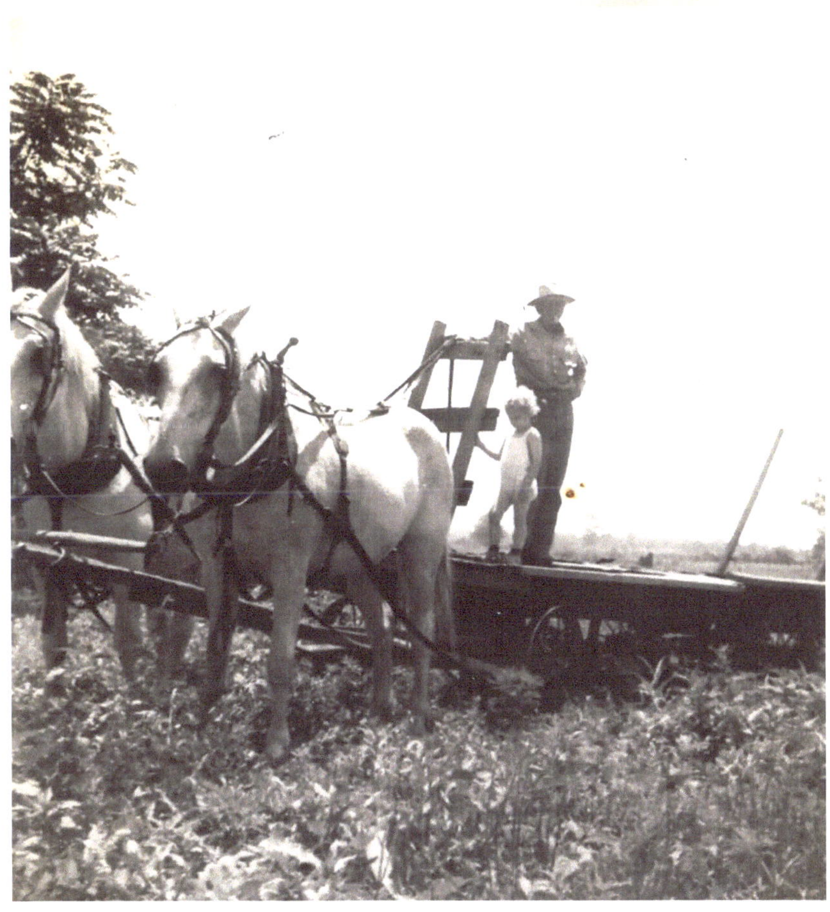

They told him the stories about pulling plows that turned over the earth. That the humans put seeds in the plowed earth to grow the hay, carrots, and apples the humans brought to us to eat.

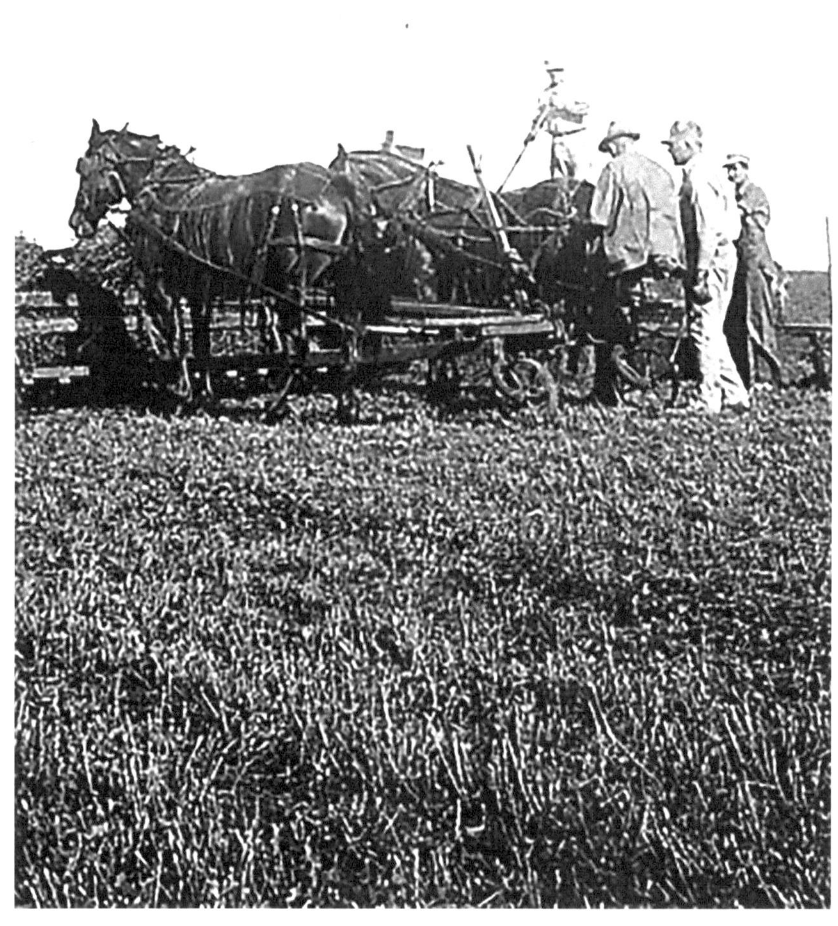

Promise's new friends told him about pulling humans in carriages, buggies, and wagons..

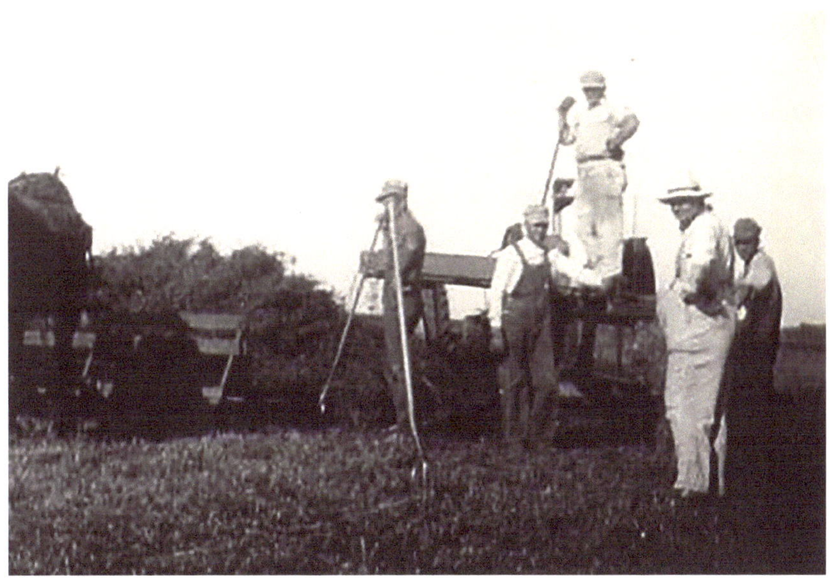

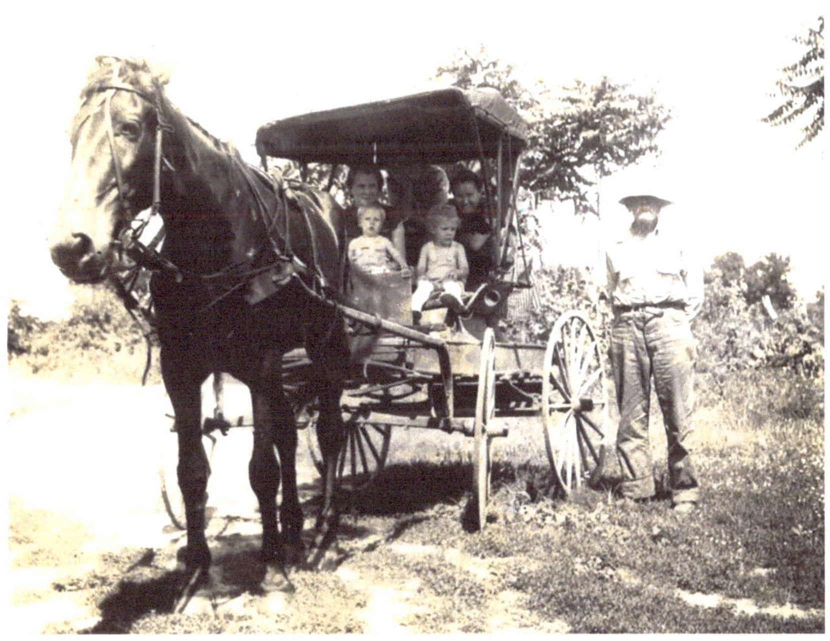

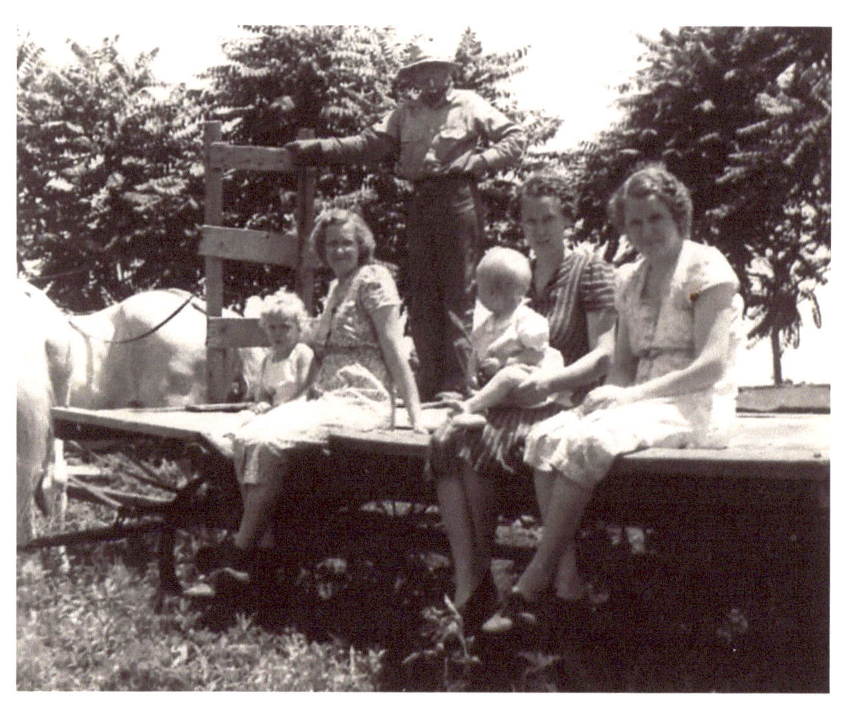

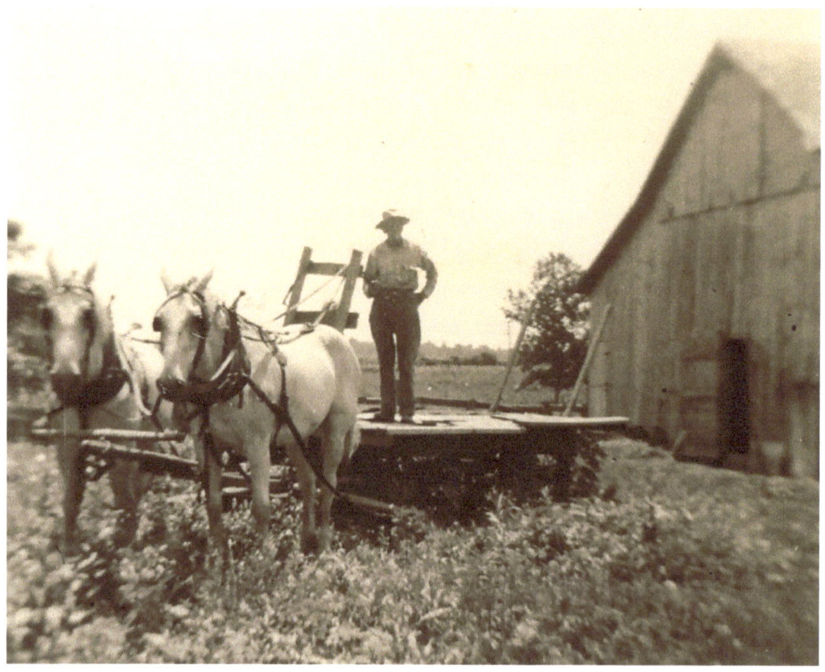

Two of the friends were brothers. They told Promise of how they were trained to work together to pull things as a team. The training to work together as a team was hard work and difficult.

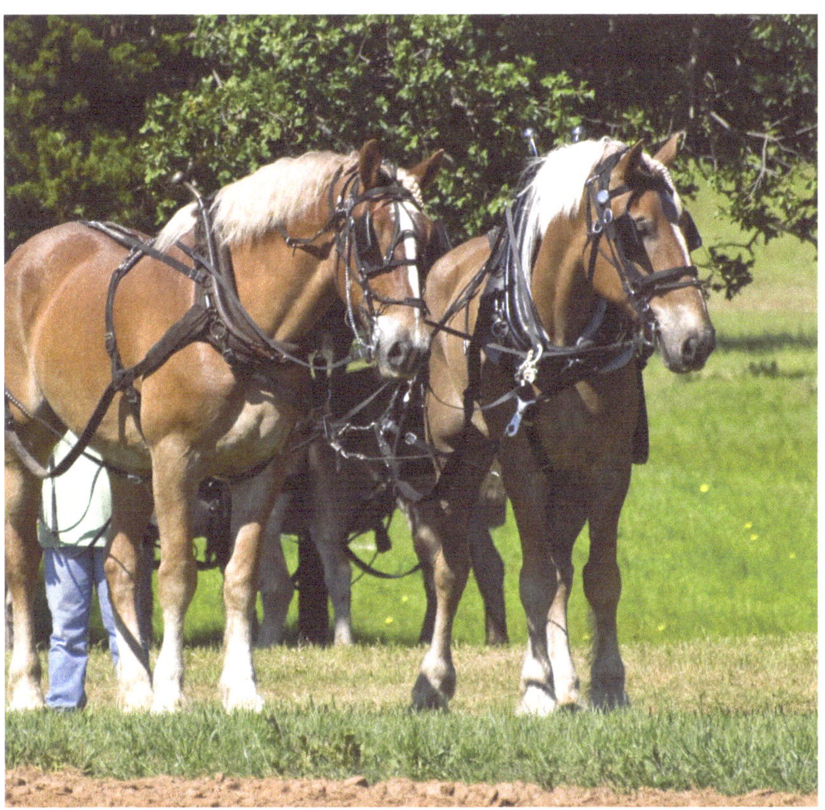

Things were made worse when the human in charge of us would get mad when we were not pulling as a team. He would hit us with what he called a whip. Once we learned to work together as a team and felt the rhythm of the trot, the team would trot proudly on the earth or a hard street. The rhythm of a team was fun, but it was still work.

Promise asked me who was his father. This was the most difficult question I had to answer. First, it was about the bad times and second, I knew that Promise would undergo a surgery to be gelded so in the near future he would not be able to breed with a mare.

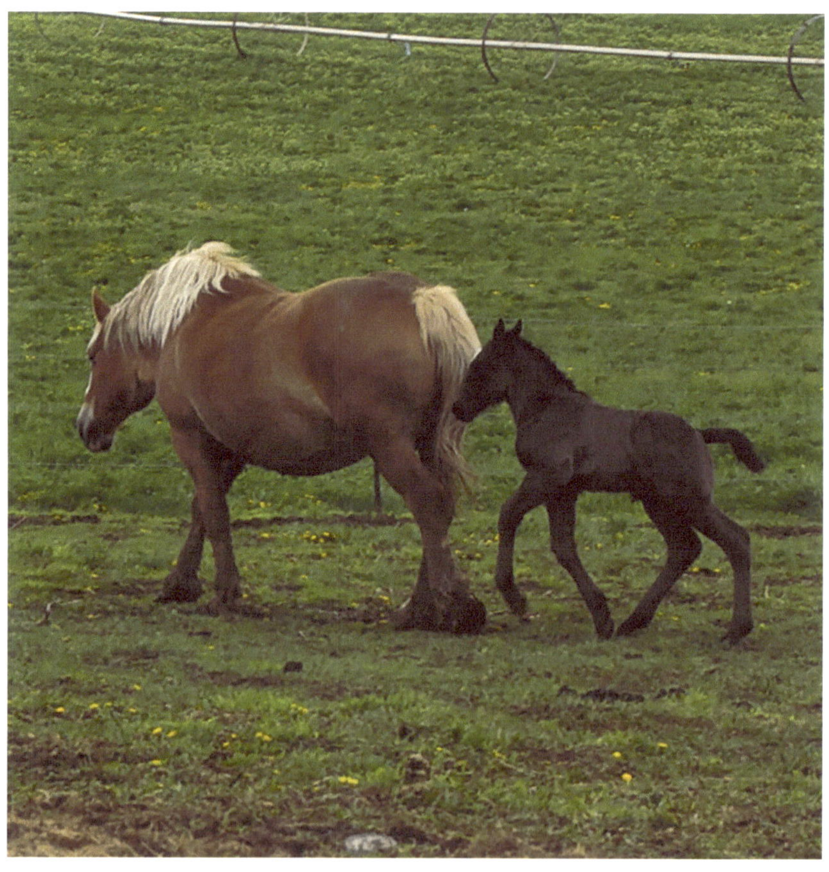

Molly Belle understood the reasoning behind the decision to geld Promise. She understood that a stallion could become violent when his hormones were strong and a female in Estrus was near.

Finally, after much pestering, she told Promise about the farm and his lost siblings.

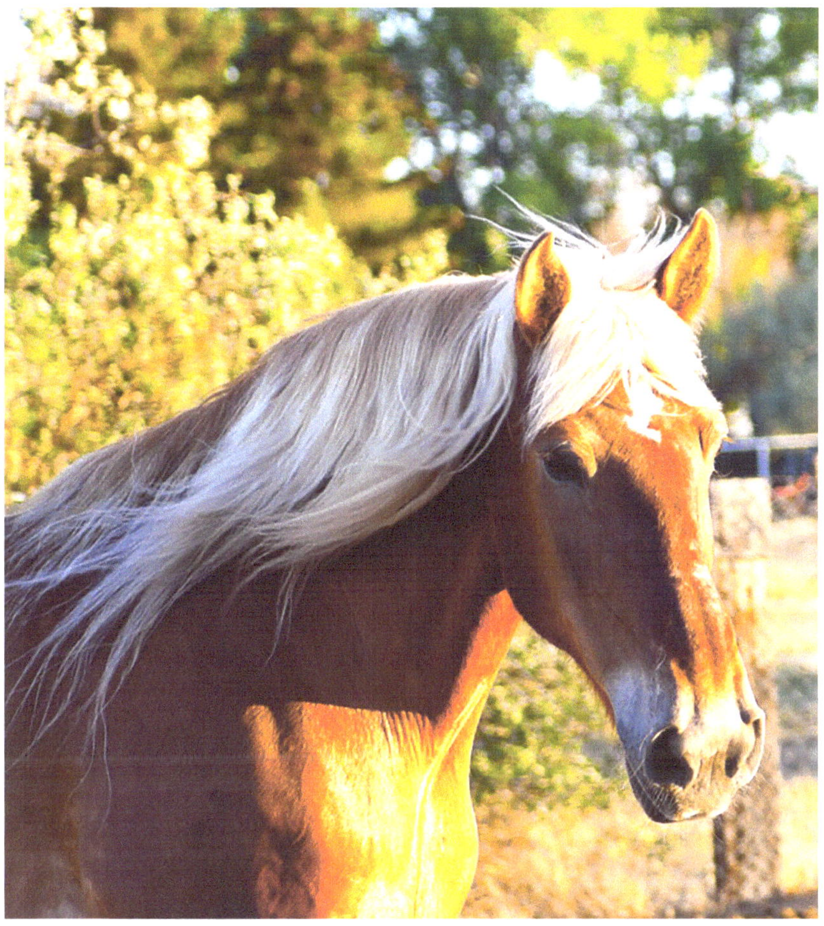

Molly Belle began her story of Promise's father: "The humans kept a few stallions on the farm as breeders. When I was able to be pregnant again, I was placed in a fenced in special breeding pasture all by myself. Eventually a gate in the fence would be opened and a stallion would trot into my pasture.

There was not much fussing around as we both knew our job.

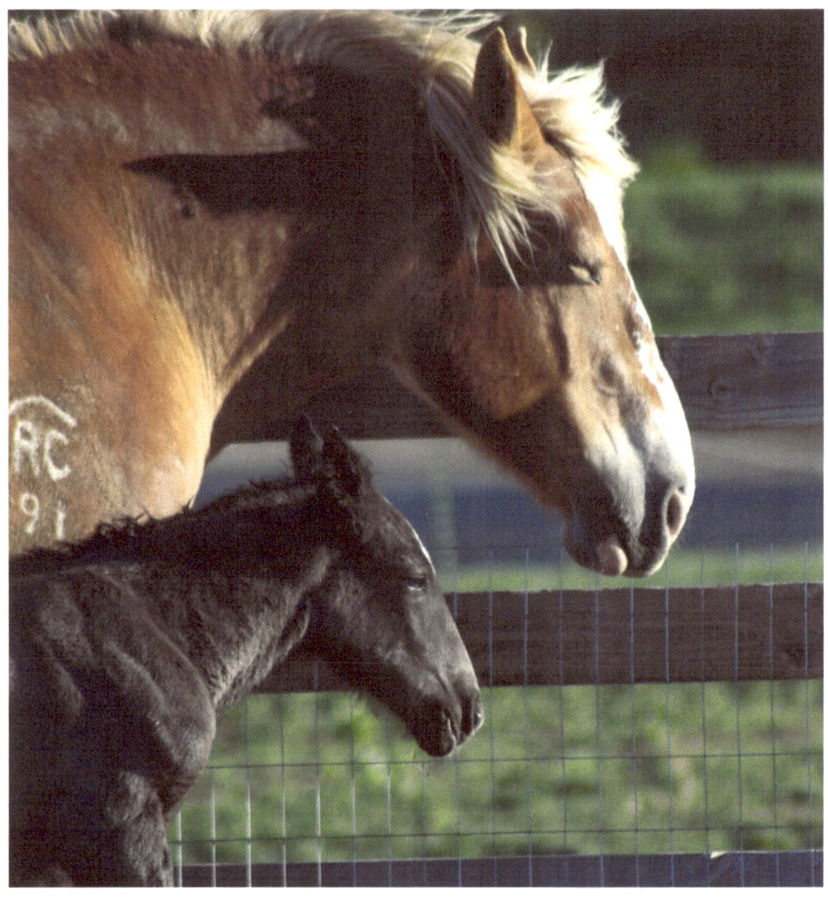

Promise was smart and asked: "Since the humans controlled the breeding, how come they did not know that a stallion was let into your pasture?"

Molly Belle finally told her foal the love story behind the birth of Promise.

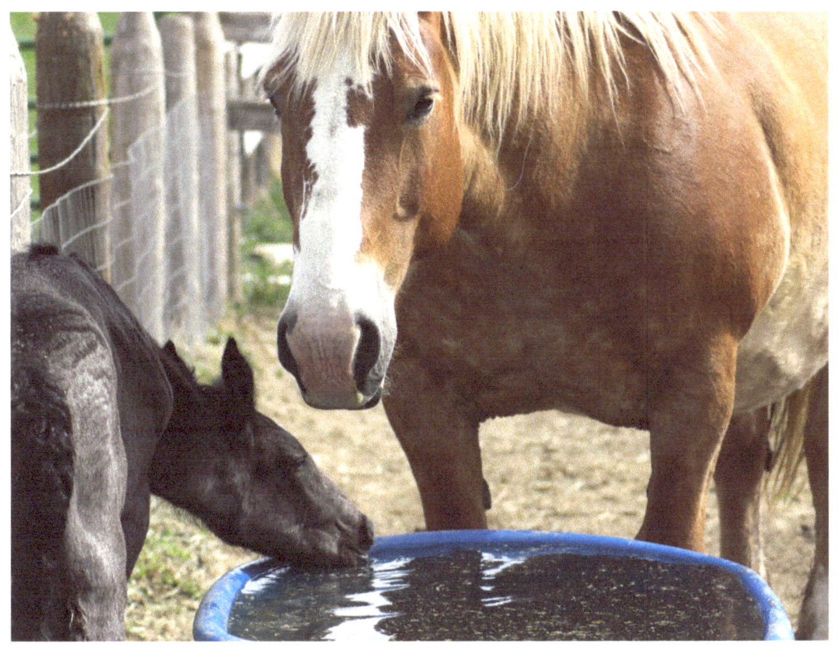

"Over the years that I was on the farm, it seemed that the humans always let the same stallion into my pasture. His name was Squire."

"The owners were always happy as it was just a short time before I became pregnant. Squire and I became lovers and it was fun to be with him if only for a little while. So, the humans thought, why change a successful formula. As time went by, they knew that at some breeding cycle that I would not be a useful urine producer to the humans and they would send me away. Squire and I developed a plan. He understood the pain I went through with each birth and my inability of raising the foal. He also was in pain and grieved to have not been able to see his foals."

"The plan was to mate with me without the humans knowing we had mated and that I might be pregnant. When they introduced Squire into my pasture I would outwardly reject him. I would keep rejecting him until the humans determined that I was not going to mate and that I was too old to be of value and would send me away."

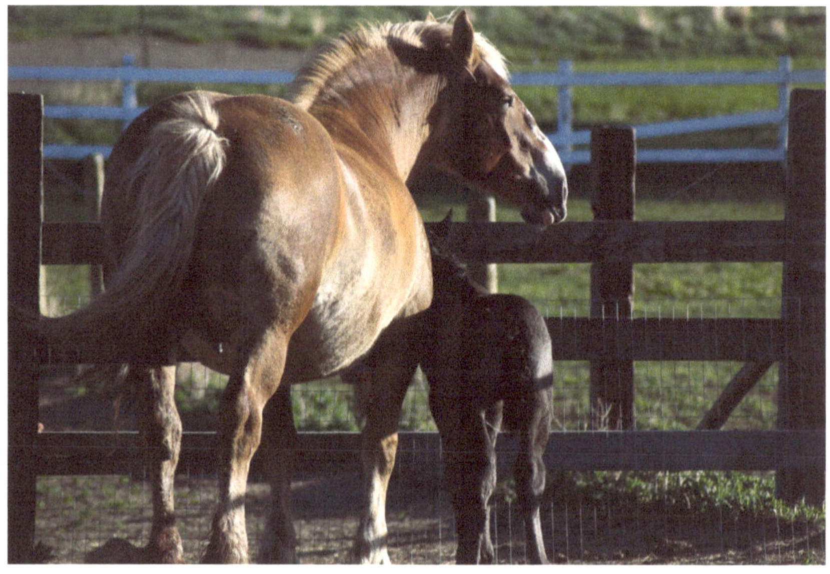

By this point in my story, Promise was snuggling up to me listening to me tell the story of his father. Promise whinnied: "Mom, please go on."

I went on: "Last warm season I was in my pasture resting after giving birth to my 10th foal. I knew that my hormones were active, and that I was in Estrus and capable of becoming pregnant. It was time that the humans would usually open the gate for Squire."

"We muzzled across the fence and decided to implement our plan."

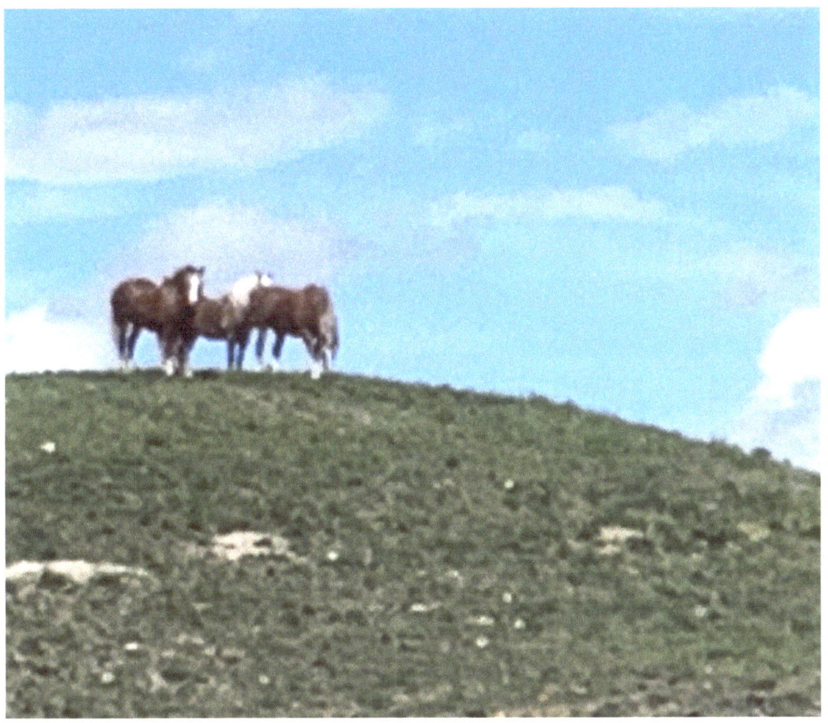

"The humans opened my gate and Squire proudly trotted into the pasture to do his duty. He was a beautiful stallion and I really loved him. I forced myself to run away and make him chase me. Every time Squire got near me I would run away. The humans were watching."

"After two days of Squire trying to mate with me, the humans stopped opening the gate and there was silence in my pasture. The humans had given up on me."

"On the night of the third day of silence, I was awaken by the sound of the gate to my pasture opening."

"I looked around. In the darkness. There was a slight breeze, and the odor of Squire was in the air. I knew that this was going to be a wonderful night and it would be the last time I saw Squire."

"He nudged me and we silently mated. Squire nudged me again in a silent good-bye and went back to his pasture nudging the gate closed. We both knew that I wanted to keep a foal. We knew of no other way."

Promise moved closer to his mother as proof of his understanding of my story of the bad times and the beauty of mating with his father, Squire.

The days of Promise turned into years. He grew and grew until he was 18 hands (6') tall and weighed 2,000 lbs. He almost became as tall as Knight of Dreams.

Promise never challenged Knight for being the leader of the herd. I had told Promise about Knight's welcoming me to join the herd.

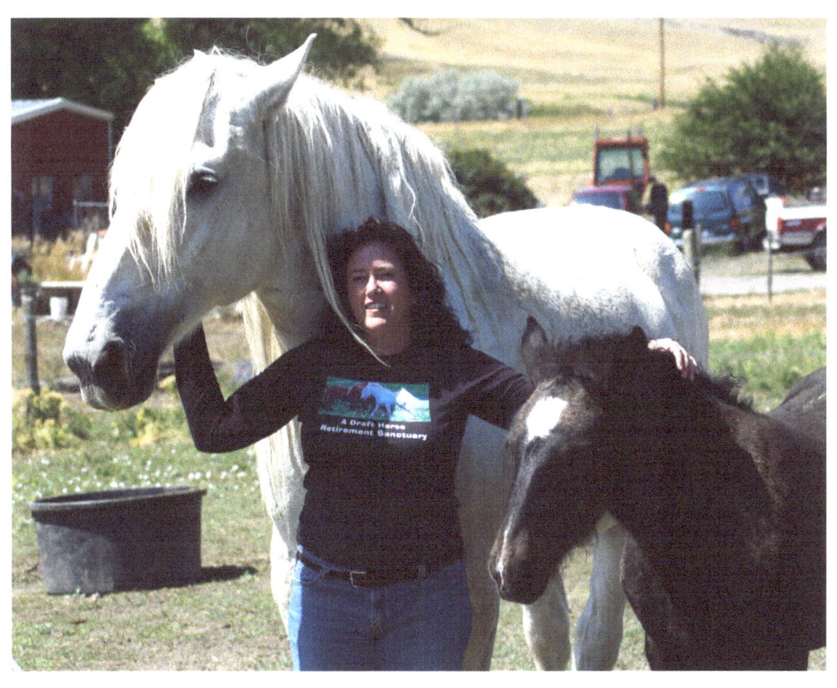

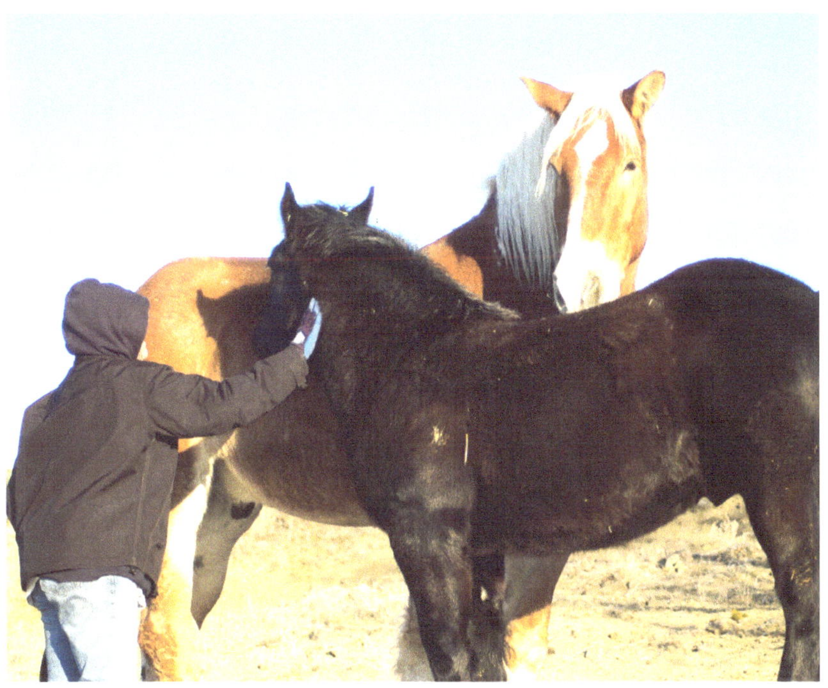

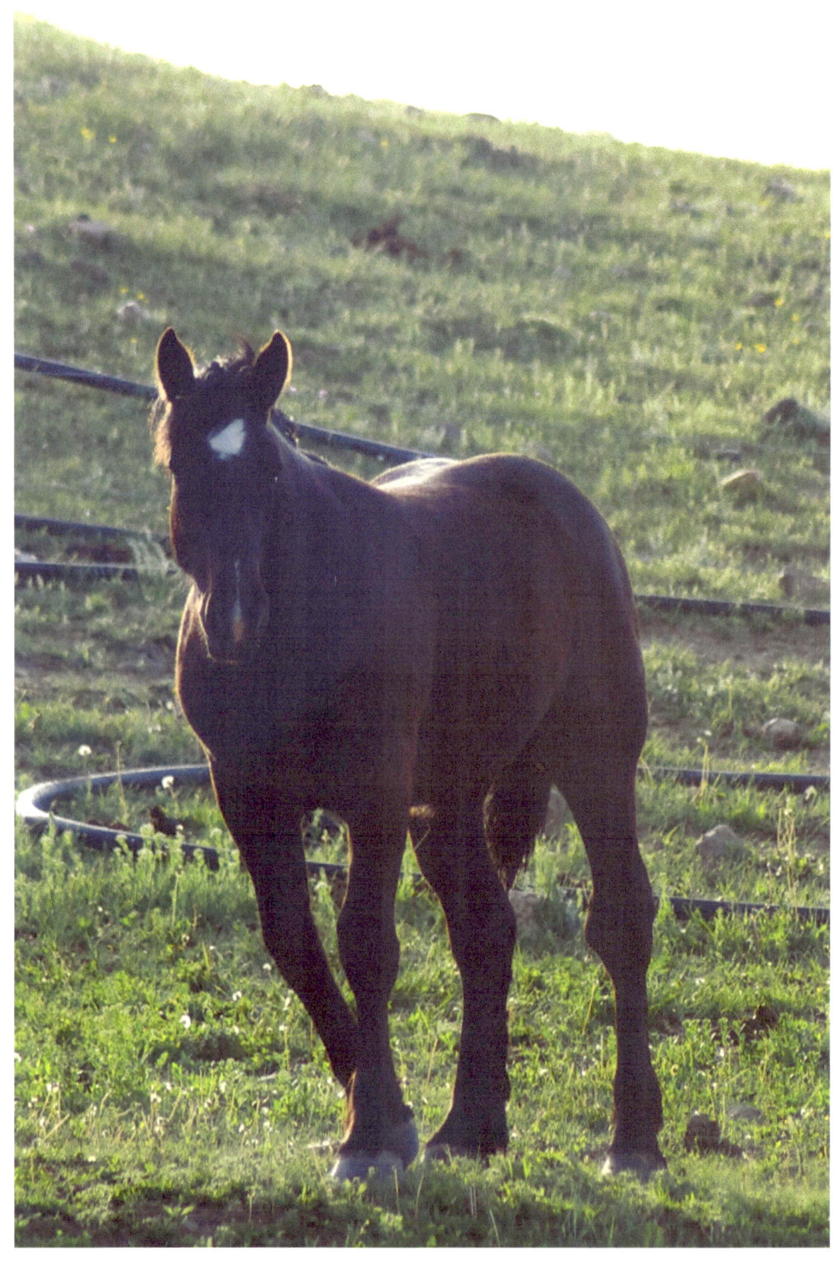

IN SUCH A SHORT TIME IT WAS OVER

Promise did not have time to be a leader. He was having too much fun. He would run with the wind. Trotting up the high hills of the pasture to survey his Paradise Valley domain.

Molly Belle was so proud of Promise. He was now a colt and growing fast into a full-grown horse and a friend to the herd. He was growing so fast that it amazed Molly Belle and the rest of the herd. We knew that all the friends had a teaching role in Promise's growth and wisdom.

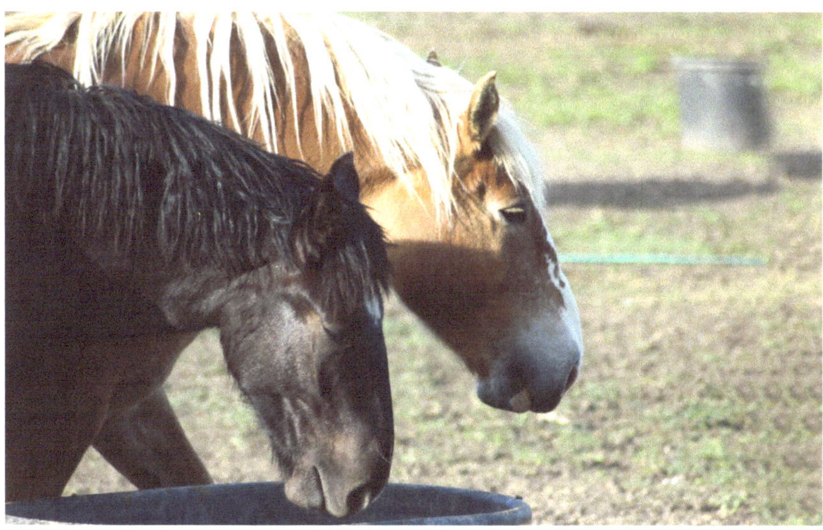

The best part of the Promise story was that he only grew old in wisdom and not in playfulness. One of his tricks was running at the herd and scatter them disrupting their sedentary life of growing old in peace.

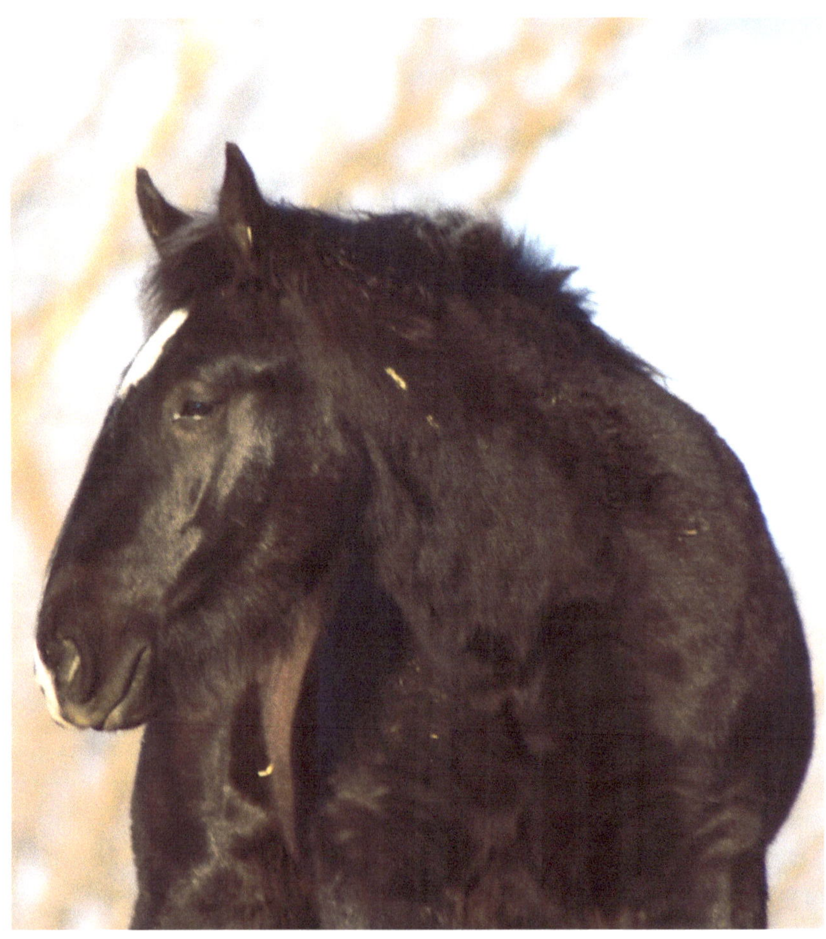

It was funny to see how he frightened humans. They would see Promise playing or grazing on the other side of the pasture. They would start to walk towards him. His head would be down nibbling grass. He would periodically raise his head to look around to note what was happening. Then when the human was still a long way off, he would raise his head and charge the human at full speed.

The human did not know quite what to do.

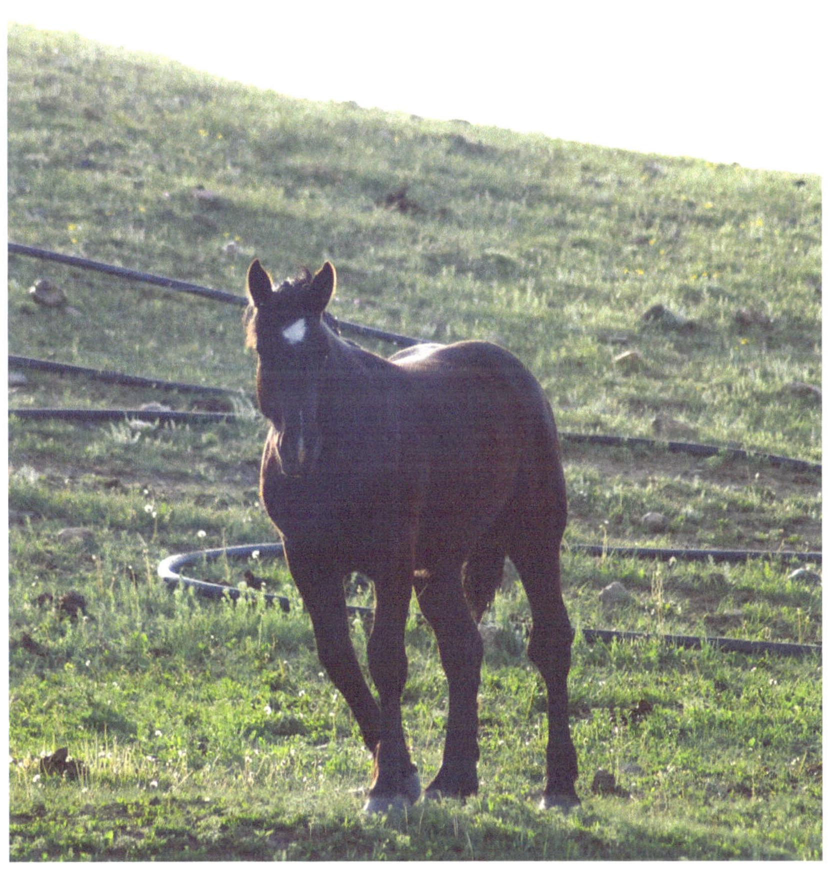

The human would stop walking, turn around and run like they were being chased by the spirit of the devil. Promise would never chase the humans once he saw them start to run, he would gradually come to a halt, turn, and nonchalantly walk away and start grazing again.

The human would eventually turn to see if Promise was still pursuing. To their surprise, Promise had his back turned and was pleasantly grazing.

This event was witnessed by the herd and there was a great deal of whinnying by everyone. It was the main event of the day.

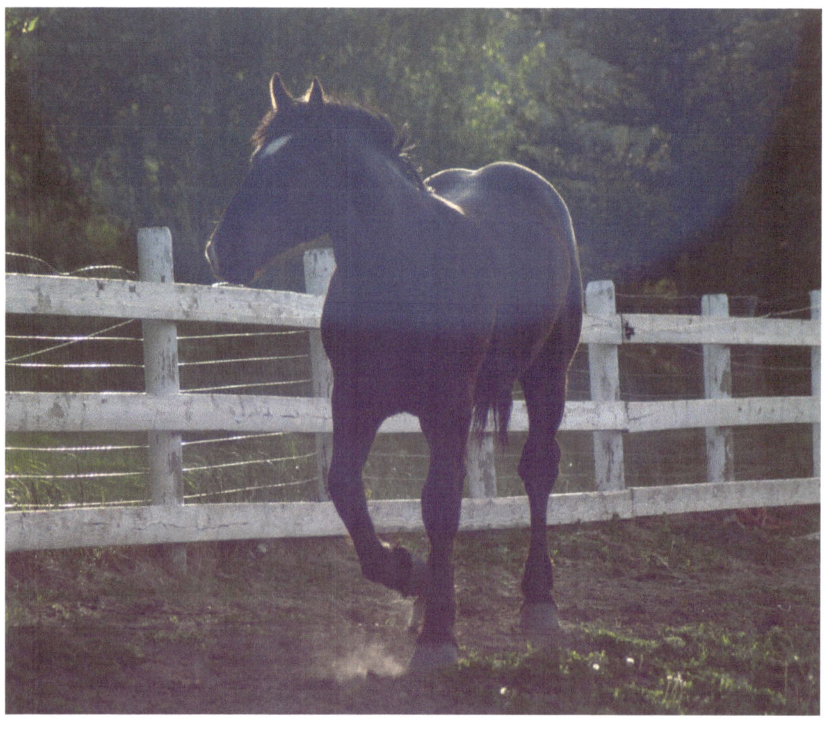

There were humans that knew Promise and the charging trick. These knowledgeable humans would approach Promise and when they saw him start his charge they would stop and look right at him. He would continue his charge until he was ten feet from the human. He would then put on the brakes with his front feet and come to a dusty five-foot stop.

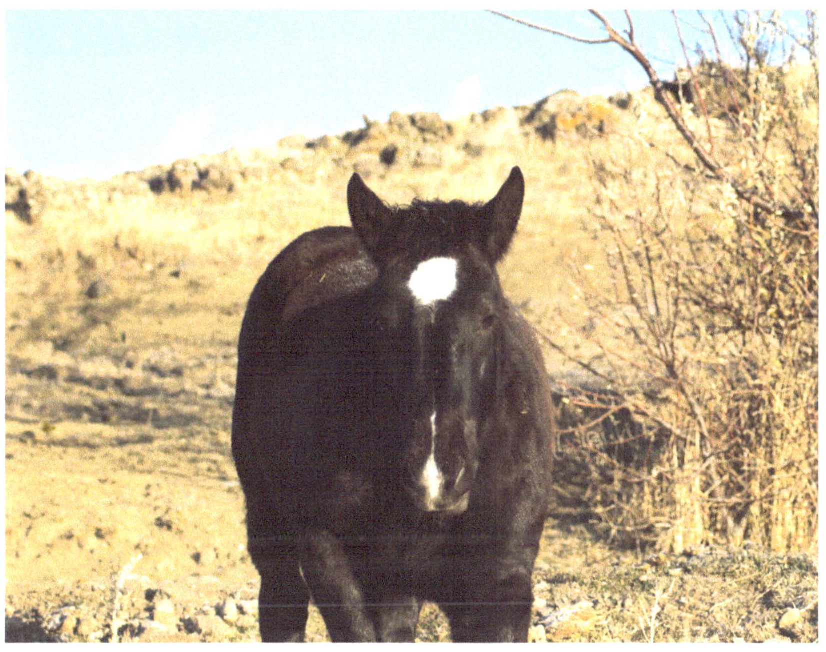

The human would stroke his head and Promise would let out a loud whinny quickly joined by choruses from the herd.

I spoke of the main event of the day. Well, Dr. Deb had a big party every year. She called it the MANE EVENT. Get it? (Molly Belle whinnied at her own humor).

The MANE EVENT would be held during warm weather. It always seemed that the activity started right after I had shed my winter coat. Dr. Deb would have other humans put up a large white tent to keep the hot sun from shinning down on their party. Humans would be walking around the pasture and visiting with us. Some would have a brush. We would enjoy being brushed and groomed.

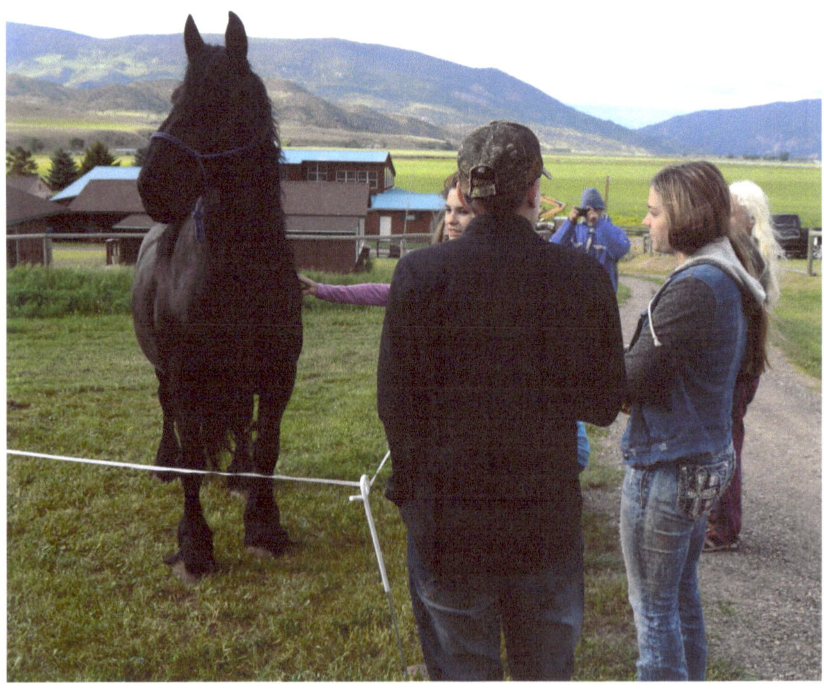

There were so many human happy and friendly odors. Of course, Promise was right in there with the crowd. He acted as though he was one of the human groups and they loved that he was so friendly.

Dr. Deb also held parties other than the MANE EVENT. Smaller groups of Humans came to visit and see us. They would bring us apples, carrots, and sometimes melons. It was a fun time for the herd and especially for Promise. He was the most energetic of all the friends and many times he would make the friends a little annoyed at his actions.

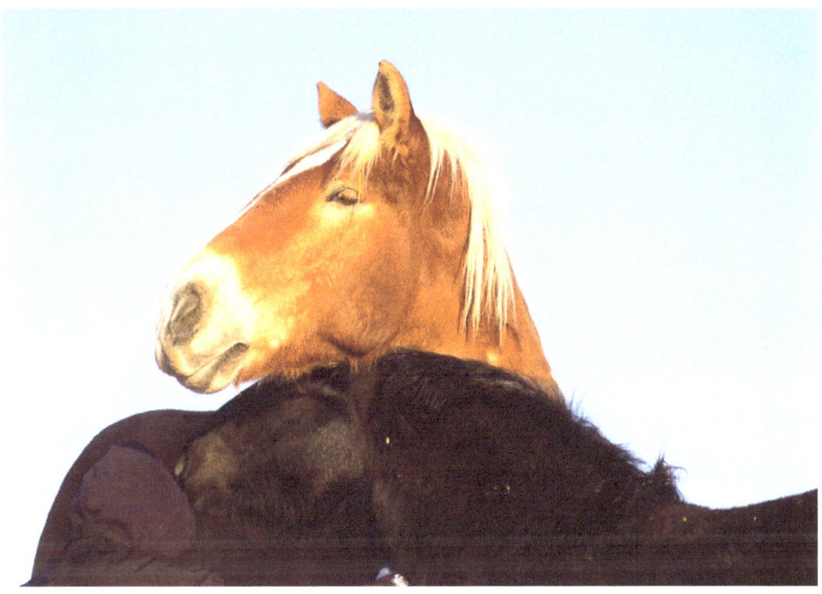

The humans would be standing on a deck that was raised off the ground and high enough that their hands holding the apple was at the level of our mussel. Dr. Deb knew if the apple was dropped, we could not see well. The humans wanted to give us the apple by holding them out in their hands so we could take it from them without biting their hand. We did not want to bite the hand that fed us. (Molly Belle gave another small whinny).

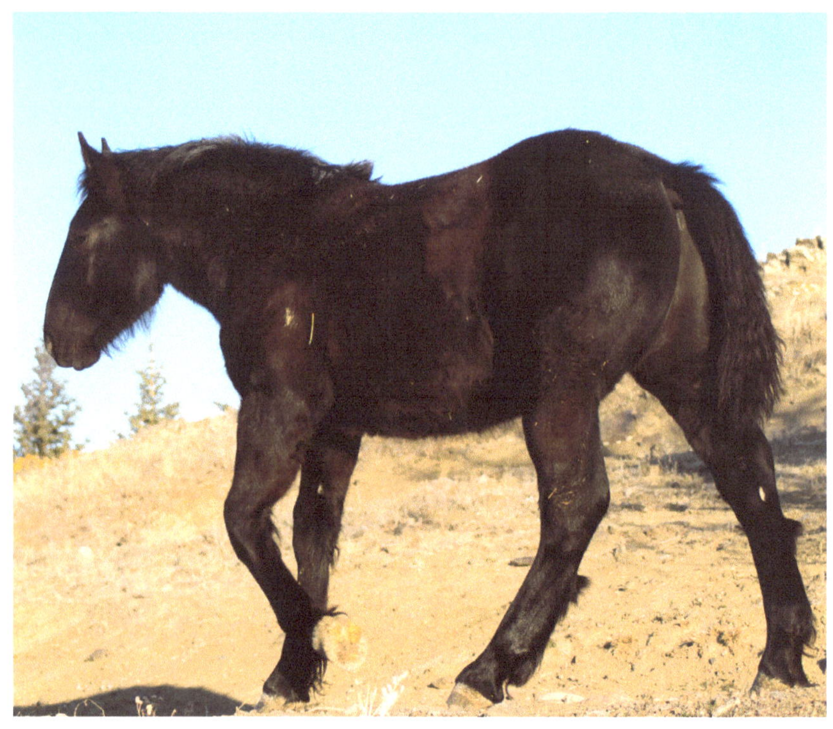

Promise was a growing colt and figured that he should have the bulk of the apples and carrots. He always planned to be the first to recognize that humans were arriving and were about to start handing out apples.

Promise would start his "charge" routine and the friends would give him room to proceed. The friends would receive a face full of the dust he kicked up in his charging process. The friends would move to one side and let him into the line of humans and then proceed to stand beside him to receive their share of the apple bounty.

There was another horse in another pasture that was not part of our herd. Her name was Tinker Bell. She used to stand on the other side of the pasture fence and watch us being fed the apples. One time it seemed that Promise knew that Tinker Bell would surely like an apple. Some of the apples had dropped to the ground and they seemed to just be lying there while the friends ate from the hands of the humans.

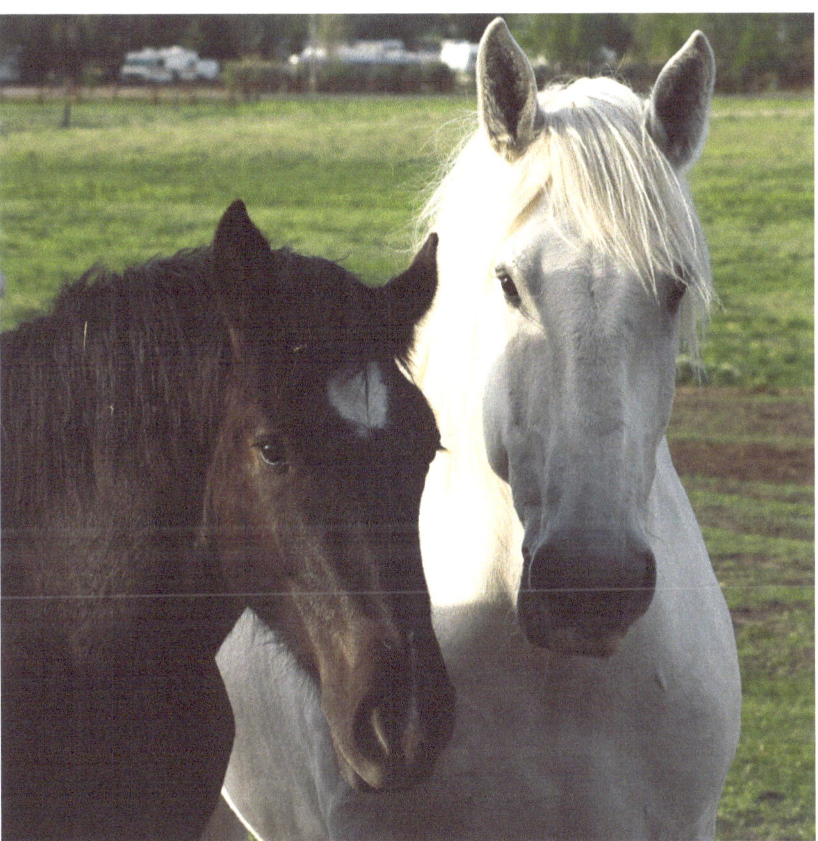

An apple was lying close to the fence but not close enough for Tinker Bell to reach. Promise walked over to the apple and kicked it under the fence into Tinker

Bell's pasture. He then strutted back to the deck and pushed aside a friend and began eating again.

If you weren't paying attention, and your back was turned he would kick over the feeding tanks. After the human heard the noise they would look over at Promise.

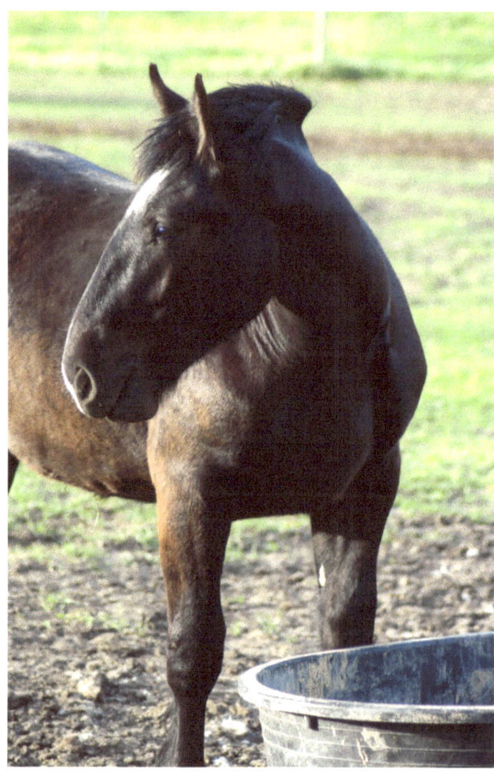

He would stare back as if saying: "Where is my food".

There were days spent walking in the Livingston 4th of July Parade. Or visiting the farmers market and watching the humans pick their food.

They would always walk over to Promise and talk to him while they were rubbing his muzzle.

Most of all he loved the days when there was an

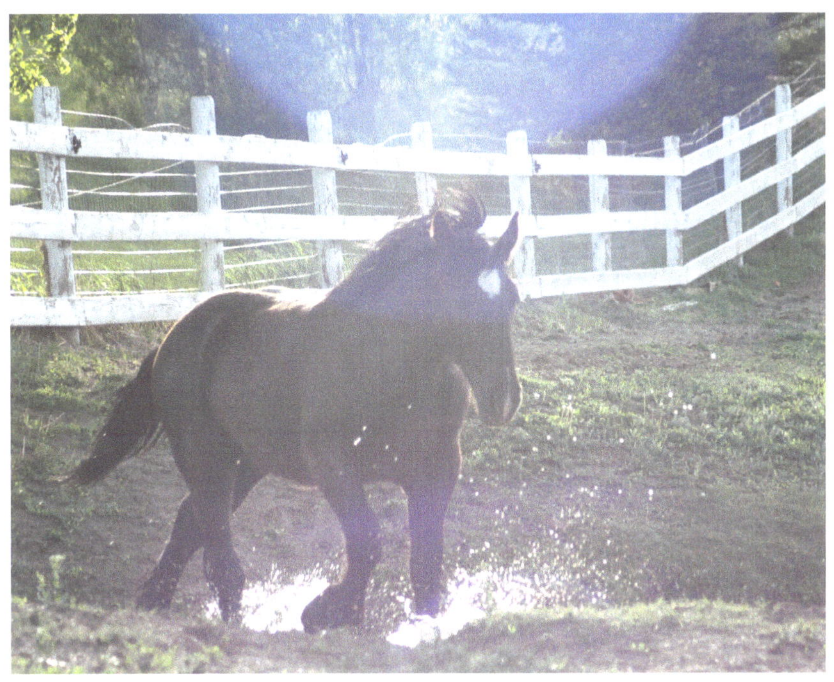

Open House and families would visit the ranch. They always brought apples and carrots. Sometimes they brought melons and Promise would kick them around like a ball.

During the Open House after I had my fill of apples

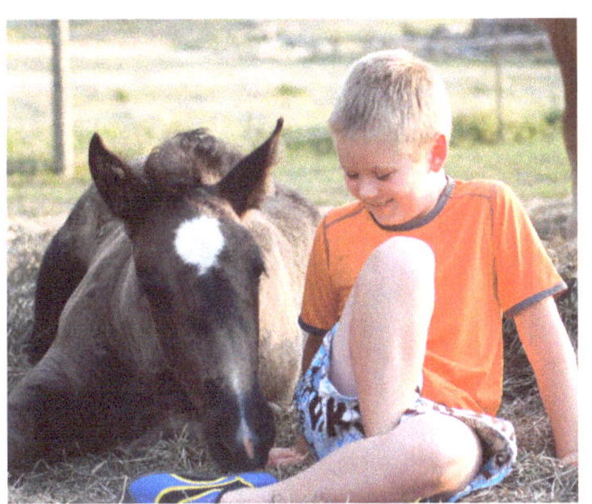

and carrots, I would stand off to one side and watch Promise have fun. He would dodge in-between the other horse friends and steal an apple that was meant for one of the other horses right out of a little girl or boy's hand. I could see our friend's reaction to this Promise mugging. Their heads would come up and swing around to nip the friend which had the nerve to steal their apple. They would see that it was Promise and relax.

At times they would whinny at Promise just to let him know that this was not within the rules of good manners.

Promise would whinny back or blow a blubber as he

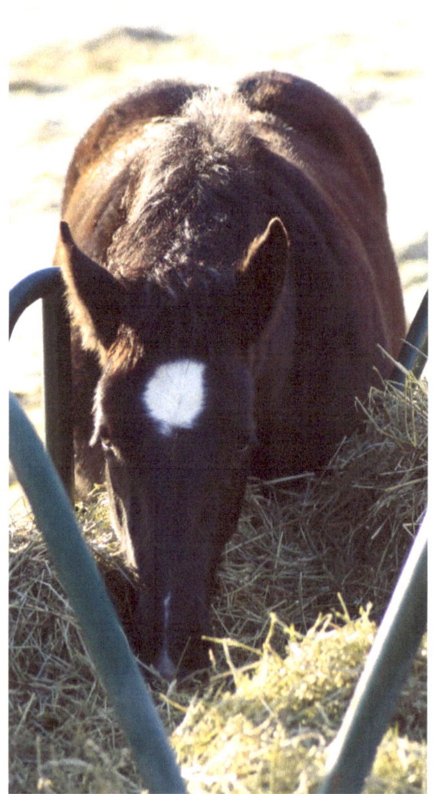

majestically pranced out of reach of the old friend's teeth. It would be only seconds when everything was back to normal.

There were always enough apples and carrots. Dr. Deb and the other ranch crew members always made sure no one went hungry

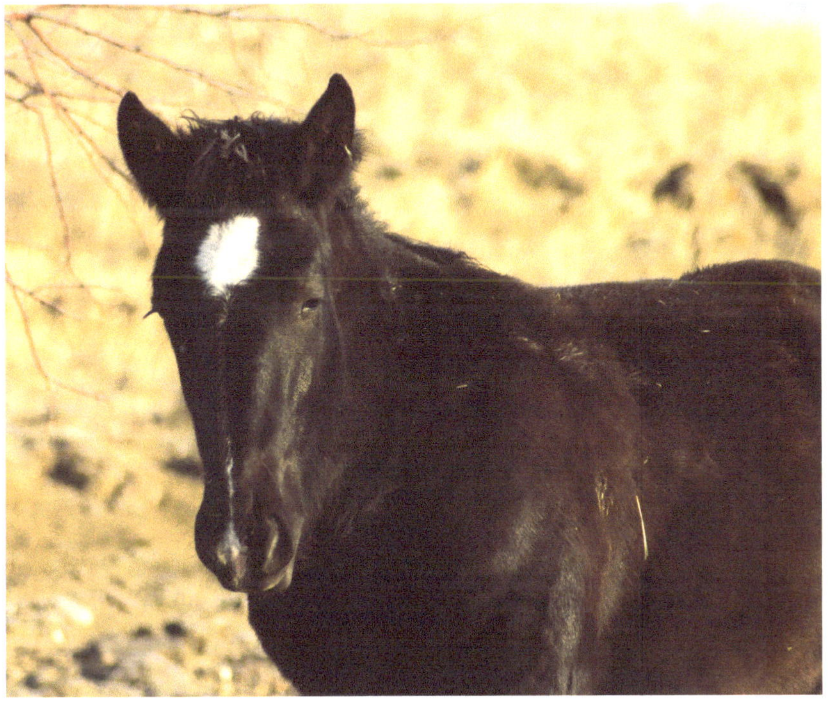

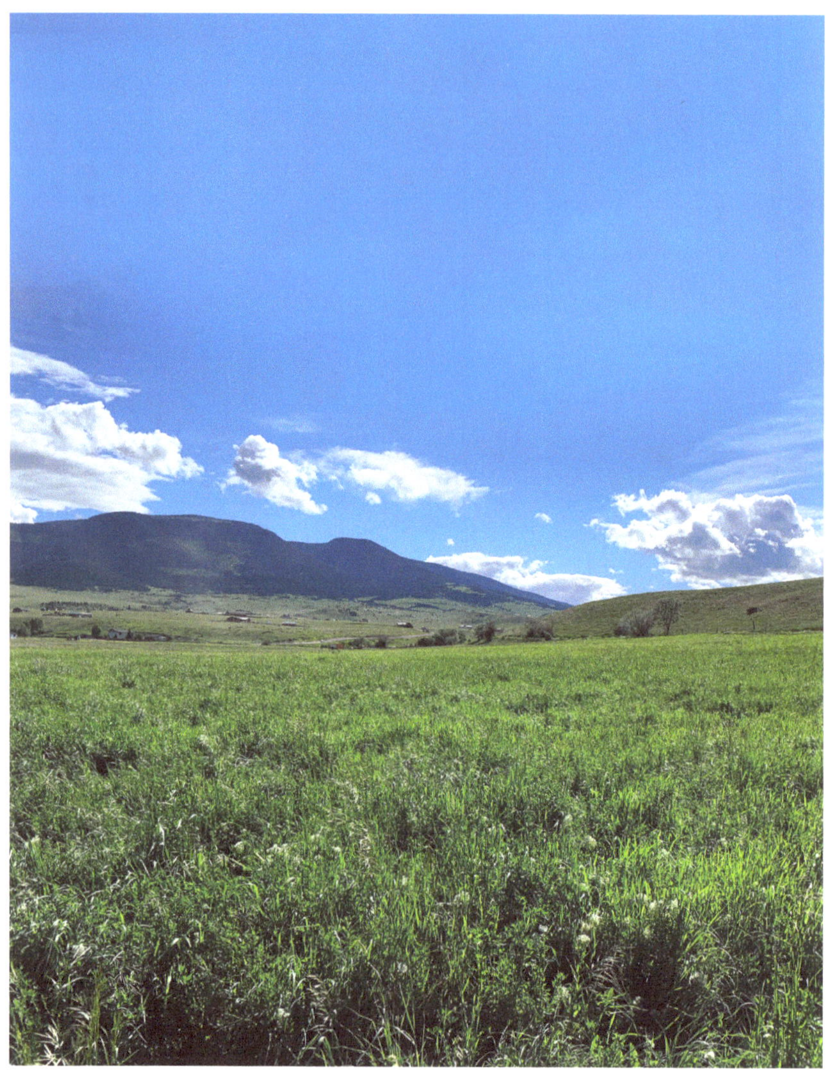

Another Promise favorite trick was to be given a juicy apple by a little boy or girl while their human stood by with a camera. Promise would wrap his large lips around the apple while the child held on so it would not be dropped. Then he would bite down on the apple and squirt juice over everyone.

"I awoke one morning to a great deal of stirring by my friends. I could feel that something was wrong and there was sadness all around me. It was a sunny morning and I had laid down to rest. I was nudged by Knight."

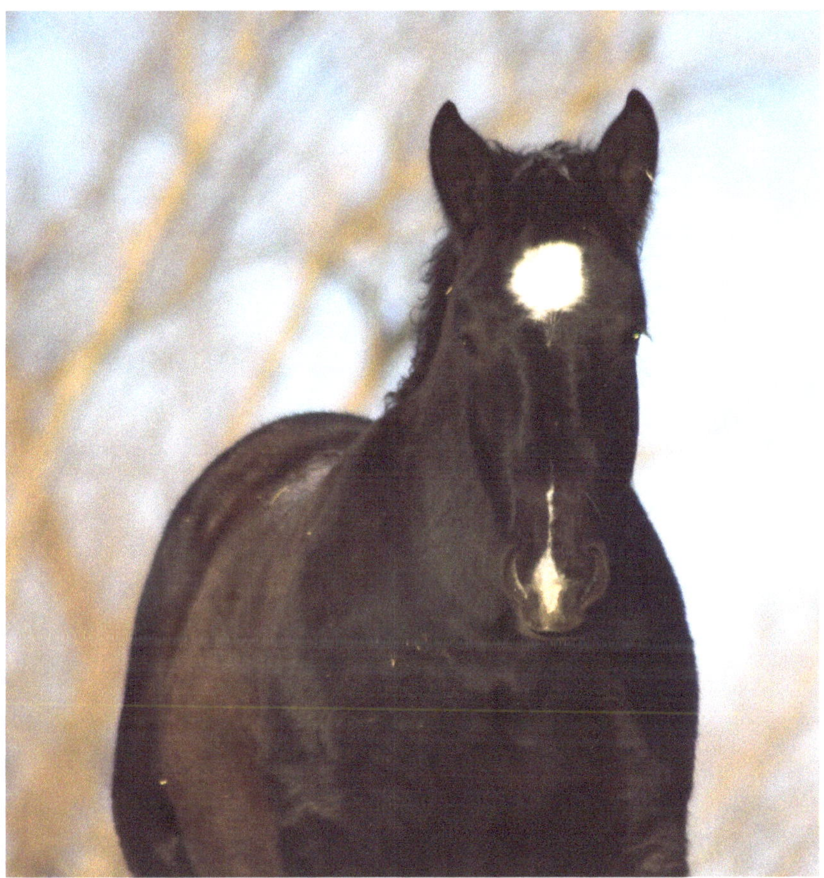

"I stood up and went out into the pasture. All my friends were standing around Promise who looked like he was sleeping. His beautiful black body adding contrast to the green grass."

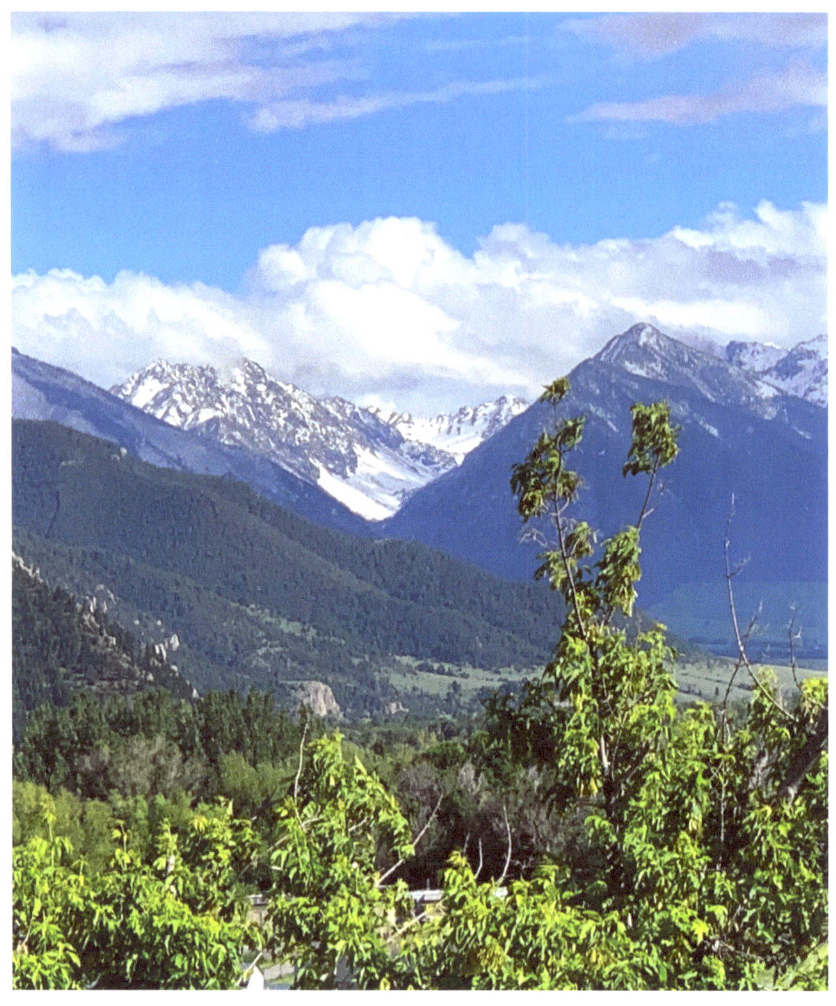

"My mind told me that I had lost my beautiful Promise. I could feel that my friends were all in mourning. There was no whinnying of happiness or joy in the pasture."

"I nudged Promise in a futile attempt of his awaking to his mother's wishes. I bowed down and placed my head next to him and cried."

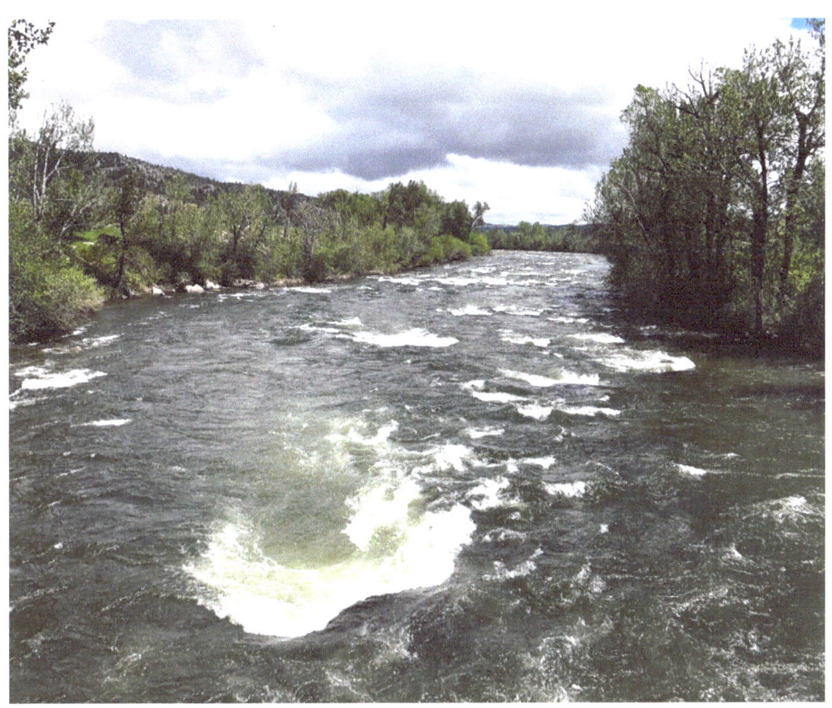

A low growl took over my total body and I knew the cause was the bad life I was forced to live while on the Premarin Farm that killed my Promise.

Promise was seven years old when the spirits took him away from me; the friends in the herd; and the humans who loved him.

Dr. Deb came to see what had happened. I knew she would feel the same sense of loss that I felt as she was Promise's human Mother. She knew that Promise had crossed over into the Light. Dr. Deb knelt down beside Promise and I could hear her as she cried human tears of sorrow.

We all gathered around Promise and mourned our loss and felt his spirit leave his body and flow to the light.

After Promise was taken away, Dr. Deb visited me, she hugged me and we both cried again. She told me that the Horse Doctor had told her that Promise had a weak heart and he had suffered a sudden heart attack.

The Horse Doctor said that Promise's weak heart was directly caused by my bad times on the PMU farm, and resulted from the many foal's that I had given birth to and lost. He was surprised that with my years of suffering I had the strength to give birth to Promise.

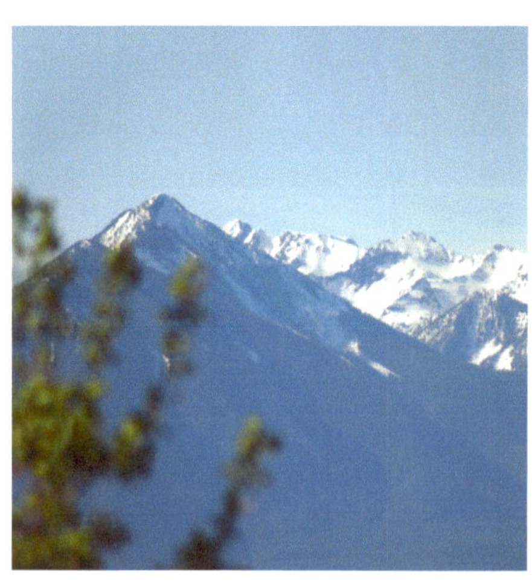

The morning continued after that sad day.

Humans would come up to me and hug me and tell me how sad it is that we had all lost Promise. He brought a happiness to the pasture that was never duplicated. Dr. Deb rescued other friends that had been on a Premarin Farm. We used to put our heads together and tell stories about the bad times.

None of the new Premarin Farm friends were pregnant when they arrived at the ranch. Some said that they had tried the same secret trick that I had accomplished but, the owners had aborted the pregnancy.

They were then sent to the Feeding Lot where, in many cases, they were saved by Dr. Deb's United in Light ranch and became my friend.

I am now a very old Mare and I feel that my time here in paradise is short. I thank the spirits, my human and horse friends, and Dr. Deb for my having seven years with my Promise. As well as the ten years I have spent living in the pastures of United in Light.

The last cold season was so very hard on me. My coat was not as warm as before. Dr. Deb paid special attention to me. I loved her for doing all she could to keep me warm and give me happy times. But, I know it is my time to cross over.

I am tired today. I don't feel like eating. I think I will lie down in the soft grass. Out of the corner of my eye I can see Dr. Deb running to me and urging me to get up. Her other human friends are running over to help.

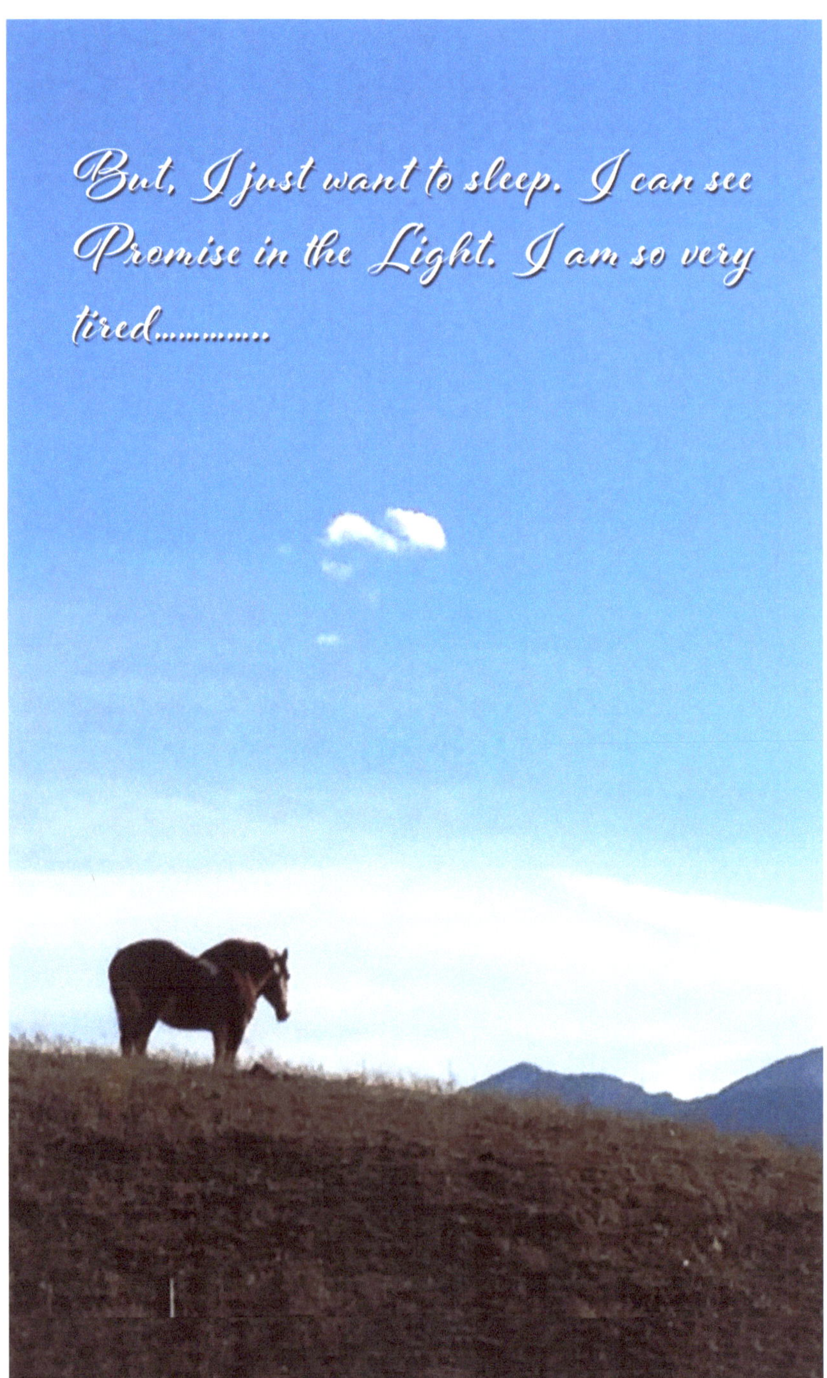

But, I just want to sleep. I can see
Promise in the Light. I am so very
tired.............

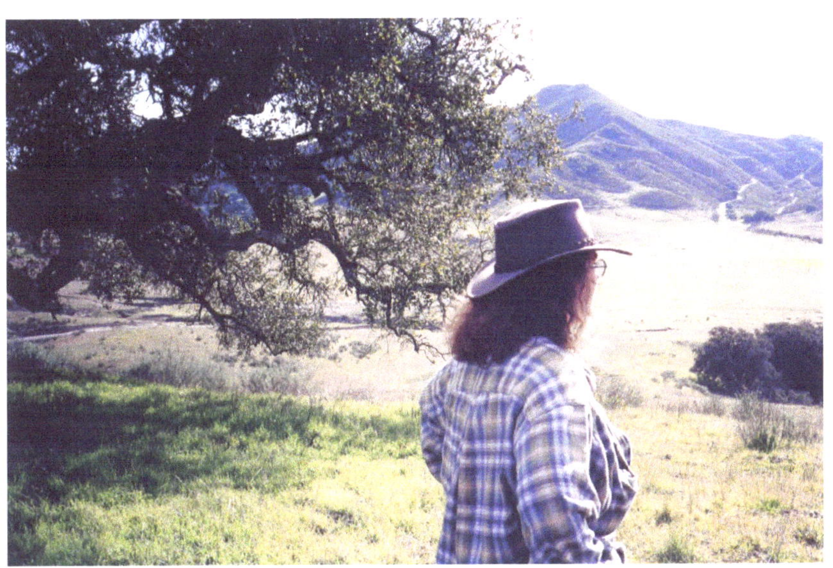

Promise is just one of the many stories about abuse and love in the world horses. With the help of the United in Light (UIL) Ranch and the Volunteers working in the Sanctuary to save draft horses from slaughter, hundreds of draft horses have been rescued by UIL or adopted by other ranches." Dr. Deborah L Derr, Doctor of Chiropractic Medicine

To learn more and to donate to this 501c3, Please go to the UIL Website: hlp://www.draftrescue.com

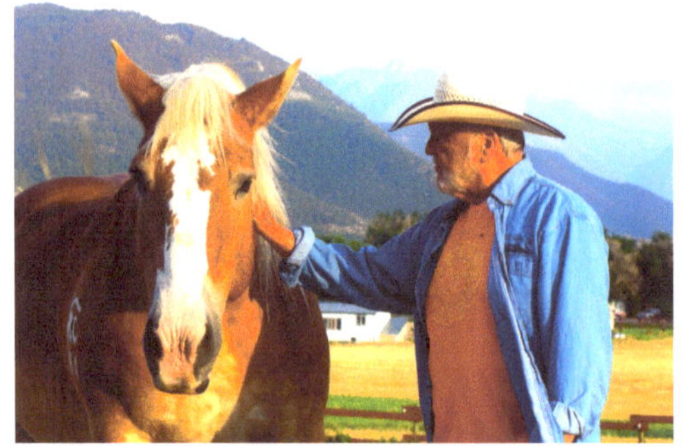

Author with Molly Belle

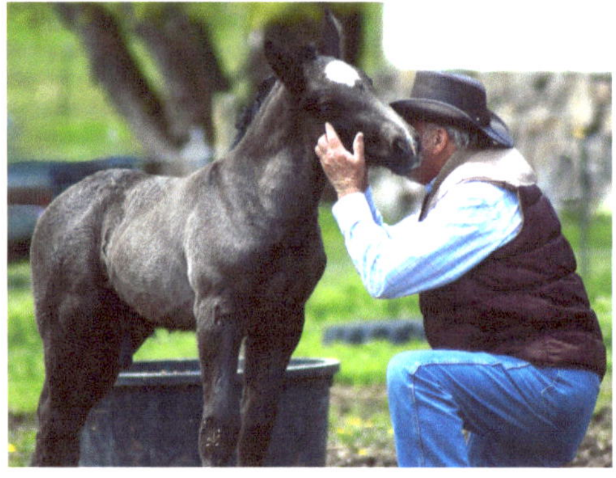

Author with Promise

The Author, Dr. John Frederick Derr, RPh, FASCP has also written a fictional novel on International Pharmaceutical Espionage titled Ancient Cure. He has also coauthored a book on An Introduction to Health Information Technology in LTPAC Settings. Both books can be purchased online at Amazon and Barnes and Noble. He has worked in healthcare at "C" Level positions for almost 60 years. More recently serving in various federal government policy committees on elderly care. He graduated from Purdue University where he was awarded Distinguished Alumnus in 2006. He is also a Retired Captain of the Line in the US Navy. He currently lives in lives in Livingston, MT.

Photographs were taken by Dr. Deborah Derr and Dr. John Derr. The black and white photographs were taken in 1940 at the author's Grandfather Bahlow's Farm in Altamont, IL. Grandfather Bahlow is Dr. Deborah Derr's Great Grandfather.

I offer gratitude and thanks to Dr. Deborah Derr for Molly Belle's story and for the writing assistance from my wife, Polly Derr, and business Assistant Deborah Cafarella.

The Sanctuary to Save Draft Horses is open to visitors with reservations and is located off Interstate 90 and State Route 89. The address is:

101 Billman Lane Livingston,
Montana 59047

Email for Reservations at:

unitedinlight@mac.com

50% of the net proceeds from the sale of this book will be donated by the Author to the Sanctuary for the Rescue of Draft Horses from Slaughter.

This book was published In June 2024 by:

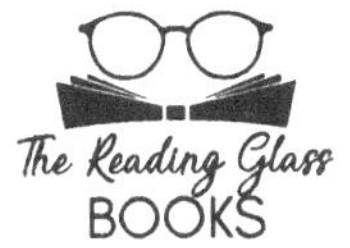

The Reading Glass Books
1-888-420-3050
www.readingglassbooks.com
fulfillment@readingglassbooks.com